Grünewald

LECTURE NOTES ON
MEDICAL STATISTICS

TO HEDVA

LECTURE NOTES ON
MEDICAL STATISTICS

AVIVA PETRIE MSc

Formerly Lecturer in Medical Statistics
Royal Postgraduate Medical School, London.
Honorary Lecturer in Medical Statistics
London School of Hygiene and
Tropical Medicine.

SECOND EDITION

BLACKWELL SCIENTIFIC PUBLICATIONS

OXFORD LONDON EDINBURGH

BOSTON PALO ALTO MELBOURNE

© 1978, 1987 by
Blackwell Scientific Publications
Editorial offices:
Osney Mead, Oxford OX2 0EL
(*Orders:* Tel. 0865 240201)
8 John Street, London WC1N 2ES
23 Ainslie Place, Edinburgh EH3 6AJ
52 Beacon Street, Boston
  Massachusetts 02108, USA
667 Lytton Avenue, Palo Alto
  California 94301, USA
107 Barry Street, Carlton
  Victoria 3053, Australia

First published 1978
Reprinted 1982, 1984, 1986
Second Edition 1987

Photoset by Enset (Photosetting),
Midsomer Norton, Bath, Avon
Printed and bound
in Great Britain

DISTRIBUTORS

USA
  Year Book Medical Publishers
  35 East Wacker Drive
  Chicago, Illinois 60601
  (*Orders:* Tel. 312 726–9733)

Canada
  The C.V. Mosby Company
  5240 Finch Avenue East,
  Scarborough, Ontario
  (*Orders:* Tel. 416–298–1588)

Australia
  Blackwell Scientific Publications
  (Australia) Pty Ltd
  107 Barry Street
  Carlton, Victoria 3053
  (*Orders:* Tel. (03) 347 0300)

British Library
Cataloguing in Publication Data

Petrie, Aviva
  Lecture notes on medical statistics.—
  2nd ed.—(Lecture notes series).
  1. Medical statistics
  I. Title
  519.5'02461   RA409

ISBN 0-632-01813-5

Contents

Preface to Second Edition

The structure and format of the second edition remain virtually identical to those of the first. However, either in response to popular demand or as a consequence of the development of statistical theory in recent years, some changes, in addition to minor alterations and supplements, have been made.

In particular, Chapter 14 of the first edition, entitled 'Computers', has been omitted. It was felt that with the rapid growth of the computer industry and the wealth of information now available in computer technology, a short chapter could not do justice to the topic. This omission is not an attempt to diminish or denigrate, in any way, an area vital to the conduct of complex statistical analyses and useful, if not imperative, for simpler procedures on small data sets. The reader is referred to any one of a number of books on computers [such as Macfarlane, P.W. (ed.) (1985) *Computer Techniques in Clinical Medicine*, Butterworths, or Longley, D. and Shain, M. (1985) *Understanding Microcomputers*, Macmillan Press] for an explanation more diverse and illuminating than the author could produce in one short chapter.

A chapter (Chapter 9) has been inserted to introduce the reader to the concepts of the analysis of variance. One- and two-way analyses of variance can be regarded as extensions, when the means of more than two groups are to be compared, to the two sample and paired t-tests described in Chapter 8. The theory underlying one- and two-way analyses of variance is developed in relatively simple terms without recourse to a discussion of mathemetical models beyond the scope of this book. Furthermore, an indication is given of the more complex applications of the analysis of variance so that the reader can become acquainted with the terminology, concepts and potential of this type of analysis.

By way of analogy, some discussion is included of the procedures for comparing more than two variances (in Chapter 5) and more than two proportions (in Chapter 10).

The chapter entitled 'Linear Regression and Correlation' (Chapter 11) has been enlarged by placing more emphasis on the extensions to simple linear regression, notably on multiple linear regression and its applications. The relevant techniques are only outlined as most rely on easily accessible computer analyses using established software for their conduct. However, it is felt that their inclusion enables the reader to appreciate the range of application and enormous scope offered to the medical research worker analysing suitable data, and to interpret the results of such analyses.

Similarly, the 'Clinical Trials' chapter (Chapter 13) has been enlarged to provide a more comprehensive account of the topic. In conjunction with it, the analysis of survival data, the development of which has been quite marked in recent years, has been expounded (in Chapter 14) within the limits imposed by the assumed non-mathematical nature of the readership.

As described in the text, a distinction is drawn between vital statistics and observational studies which provide the foundations for demography and epidemiology, respectively. To emphasise their differences, the chapter on measures of morbidity, fertility, mortality and survival is now entitled 'Vital Statistics' (Chapter 14). The contents of this chapter remain the same as those in the first edition apart from the expanded section on the analysis of survival data, mentioned previously. Furthermore, Chapter 15 has been introduced on 'Observational Studies' to provide the reader with some insight into the nature of epidemiological investigations and the statistical methods utilised therein. As with all the other additions to the book, it is felt that the reader's scope is broadened and his or her horizon's widened by its inclusion so that he or she is better equipped to understand the relevant literature and handle data in a sensible manner.

My thanks are due to Professors T. W. Anderson, Michael J. R. Healy and Geoffrey A. Rose and to Drs Michael Hills and John F. Osborn for their helpful comments and suggestions. I am also grateful to my husband, Gerald Raingold, for his patience and support and to my children, Nina, Andrew and Karen, for allowing me enough solitude to complete the manuscript.

Aviva Petrie

Preface to First Edition

Statistics is a subject which generally induces mental paralysis, occasionally contempt and, at the very least, apathy in its users. Nevertheless, statistics has been a great aid to, and is an integral part of, scientific advancement and its importance cannot be denied. Even though this is recognised by the medical student, the practising physician and the research worker, medical statistics is still to many a dark territory which should not be invaded. The problem, then, is to impart a knowledge of statistics to the learner in a manner which inflicts the minimum of pain, but, at the same time equips him or her with sufficient understanding to enable him or her to tackle statistical problems cautiously, logically and correctly.

This book is directed explicitly towards the medical applications of statistics in that some of the statistical methodology described and most of the examples included are peculiar to the medical field. It is intended to serve as a useful adjunct to lectures and fuller texts, providing the student with an outline for revision and the medical research worker with an instructive handbook.

The topics covered are those which constitute an elementary course in statistics. It is assumed that the reader is essentially innumerate and so extensive mathematical proofs are omitted. Whilst the emphasis is on methodology, theoretical considerations have not been overlooked. 'Cook-books', though welcomed by many, are often dangerous in that a lack of basic understanding can lead to erroneous analyses. For the greatest satisfaction of the greatest number, I have decided to compromise. For example, on the one hand I have tried to convey some notion of the rationale or proof underlying a statistical test, and on the other, I have paid attention to the procedural instructions to be followed when the test is performed. Furthermore, I have expressed these instructions in a standard format of seven steps so as to demonstrate that an identical logic underlies each of the many statistical tests. Somewhat unusually, I have separated worked examples from their associated theory by placing the former at the end of the appropriate chapters. In doing so, I have retained the continuity of the basic text, and yet given the reader easy access to illustrative material.

I should like to thank all those who helped and encouraged me in preparing this book. In particular I am very grateful to Professors T. W. Anderson, David F. Andrews, Peter Armitage and Michael J. R. Healy and Drs John F. Osborn and Leonard C. Petrie for their helpful comments and suggestions, and to Mrs Janice Andrews who typed the manuscript.

Aviva Petrie

Chapter 1
Introduction

Statistics

1. Statistics *are* numerical data relating to an aggregate of items (e.g. individuals) or numbers derived from the data (e.g. averages, rates).

2. Statistics *is* the science of collecting, summarising, presenting and analysing data. This analysis may lead to conclusions and subsequent decisions.

Medical statistics

The science of medical statistics embraces those techniques pertaining to the medical field. A book devoted specifically to *medical* statistics is warranted in that: (i) although the methodology of statistics is quite general, particularly at the elementary level, statistical techniques are best appreciated by the medically orientated individual if placed in a familiar context; and (ii) furthermore, specific problems arise in medicine, often because the unit of interest is a living person rather than some abstract phenomenon, object or financial consideration. Such problems merit special attention.

Classification

Broadly, statistics may be: (i) descriptive; or (ii) inferential.

Descriptive statistics

These are devices for organising data, and may be: (i) tabular; (ii) diagrammatic; or (iii) numerical.

They are merely descriptive and make no attempt to draw conclusions from the data. Descriptive statistics reduce the acquired information to a manageable size. They present a summary of the data which in their raw form are too disperse to comprehend.

1

Inferential statistics

These are concerned with drawing conclusions from the data and the conclusions drawn will influence subsequent decisions. For example, the conclusion that there is a significant difference in some measurable response between a new drug A and a standard therapy B may lead to the decision to introduce drug A on to the market.

The need for a formal methodology of statistics arises from the variability inherent in observational and experimental data. Quantities which vary are called *variables* (e.g. height, age, sex); those which do not are called *constants* (e.g. $\pi = 3.141 \ldots$, $e = 2.718 \ldots$). The latter do not require statistical study. As regards the former, the considerations of cost, time or availability do not permit study of a given variable for all individuals in a population (defined below), and so a sample (defined below) of individuals is taken. The distinction between a population and a sample is of paramount importance in statistics. An attempt is made to draw conclusions about the population on the basis of the information assimilated from the sample. The mode of reasoning is *inductive* (rather than deductive) in that the procedure is concerned with generalising from the *few* to the *many*. An alternative expression of this pathway is statistical *inference*.

Statistical inference may be subclassified into the general areas of: (i) estimation of population parameters; and (ii) hypothesis testing.

Definition of terms

The vocabulary used in statistics is not unique and yet the interpretation of a single term may vary between disciplines. To avoid confusion, it is wise to clarify the meaning of the following terms which form the basis of the language of statistics. They are loosely defined in an attempt to promote understanding and, as such, may extend over stringent mathematical boundaries.

Variable

This is a quantity which varies such that it may take any one of a specified set of values. It may be measurable (e.g. the value in mm Hg of the variable, systolic blood-pressure) or non-measurable (e.g. the 'value' male or female of the variable, sex).

Variables may be further subclassified according to their scale of measurement, as indicated in Fig. 1.1.

It should be noted that there is a graded relationship between the scales of measurement in that a particular scale possesses the characteristics of those scales to the left of it in Fig. 1.1, in addition to the specific characteristics defining that scale; e.g. the interval scale has the characteristics of nominal and ordinal scales of measurement. .

Observation

Strictly, this is an event which is seen to occur. A number, expressed as the value of a variable, is usually assigned to the event, and this is the measurement. Commonly, the term 'observation' is an expression of both the event and the measurement.

Observational unit

The source which imparts the value(s) of the variable(s) is known as the observational unit. It may be an individual item (e.g. an object, person, characteristic or event) or it may be a collection of items (e.g. a household, litter or set of symptoms). The term 'individual', not necessarily in the human context, often replaces the cumbersome 'observational unit'.

Data

These are the set of values of one or more variables recorded on one or more observational units.

Population

This is any finite (e.g. the babies born in England in 1977) or hypothetical (e.g. the babies who will be born in England in 1997) collection of observational units. The term population is used in its broadest sense and does not necessarily refer to a collection of living organisms.

Sample

This is a part of a population, generally selected so as to be representative of the population in the variable(s) under study.

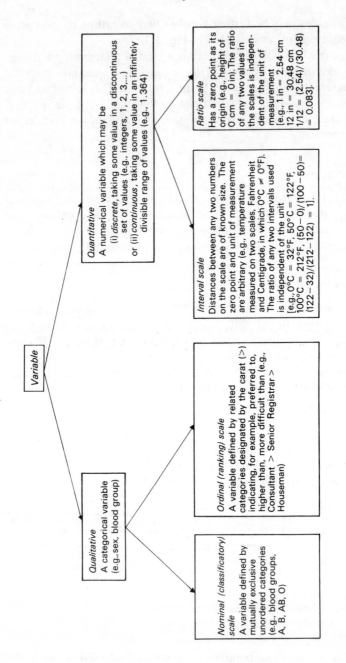

Fig. 1.1 Classification of variables.

Parameter

This is a summary value which in some way characterises the nature of the population in the variable(s) under study. Often, it is a mathematical function of the population values of the variable(s) (e.g. the population mean, the population correlation coefficient). It should not be confused with the term 'variable'.

Statistic

This is a summary value calculated from a sample of observations, usually but not necessarily as an estimator of some population parameter. Often the distinction between 'parameter' and 'statistic' is ignored and the term 'parameter' is used for both, perhaps qualified by the word population or sample. This practice should be avoided.

Notation

Statistics makes use of mathematics and thus utilises algebraic notation as an expression of its elements and methodology.

Index notation

In general terms,

> x is a symbol denoting a particular variable (e.g. age, height, or blood count).
> x_i is the symbol denoting the ith value of the variable x.
> i in x_i is the *subscript*, suffix or *index* of x.

If n observations are taken on the variable x, then i can take any one of the values $1, 2, \ldots, n$. Commonly, a single observation is referred to as x_i. Clearly, any letter other than i, such as j or k, could be used.

The set of n values of the variable x is thus the set $(x_1, x_2, \ldots, x_n)$ where

> x_1 = value of the first observation
> x_2 = value of the second observation
> .
> .
> .
> x_n = value of the nth observation.

This set is sometimes written as $(x_i; i = 1, 2, \ldots, n)$; in words, it is the set of n values of the variable x, a single value being x_i, i extending over the range of values from 1 to n. The various x_i's are not necessarily or even usually arranged in order of magnitude.

Summation notation

The summation of a set of values is an operation that occurs so frequently in statistics, that a symbol, Σ, the Greek capital letter 'sigma', is used for it. The symbol $\sum\limits_{i=1}^{n} x_i$ denotes the sum of all the x_i's from $i = 1$ to $i = n$, i.e.

$$\sum_{i=1}^{n} x_i = x_1 + x_2 + \ldots + x_n.$$

The range of values taken by the suffix is indicated above and below the summation sign. Thus

$$\sum_{i=3}^{5} x_i = x_3 + x_4 + x_5.$$

When no confusion can result, usually when the suffix assumes all values in its range, then the sum is commonly abbreviated to $\sum x$, $\sum x_i$ or $\sum\limits_{i} x_i$.

The following examples illustrate the use of Σ where x and y are two variables and a is a constant.

1. $\displaystyle\sum_{i=1}^{n} x_i y_i = x_1 y_1 + x_2 y_2 + \ldots + x_n y_n.$

2. $\displaystyle\sum_{i=1}^{n} (x_i + y_i) = x_1 + y_1 + x_2 + y_2 + \ldots + x_n + y_n$

$$= x_1 + x_2 + \ldots + x_n + y_1 + y_2 + \ldots + y_n$$

$$= \sum x_i + \sum y_i.$$

3. $\displaystyle\sum_{i=1}^{n} ax_i = ax_1 + ax_2 + \ldots + ax_n$

$\qquad = a(x_1 + x_2 + \ldots + x_n)$

$\qquad = a \displaystyle\sum_{i=1}^{n} x_i.$

4. $\displaystyle\sum_{i=1}^{n} a = a + a + \ldots + a$

$\qquad = na.$

Product notation

Whereas $\sum$ represents the sum, the Greek capital letter 'pi', $\prod$, is the symbol used to denote the product of two or more quantities.

The use of the suffix, i, with $\prod$ is identical to that with $\sum$. Thus $\displaystyle\prod_{i=1}^{n} x_i$ denotes the product of all the x_i's from $i = 1$ to $i = n$, i.e.

$$\prod_{i=1}^{n} x_i = (x_1)(x_2)(x_3)\ldots(x_n).$$

Ordered series notation

If the set of n values $(x_1, x_2, \ldots, x_n)$ of a variable is arranged in increasing order of magnitude, then $x_{(i)}$ is the value of the variable whose *rank* or *rank number* (i.e. position in the scale) is i in the ordered set. Thus

$\qquad x_{(1)}$ is the smallest value; of rank 1
$\qquad x_{(2)}$ is the second smallest value; of rank 2

$\qquad .$
$\qquad .$
$\qquad .$

$\qquad x_{(n)}$ is the largest value; of rank n

and $x_{(1)} \leqslant x_{(2)} \leqslant \ldots \leqslant x_{(n)}$ (the sign $\leqslant$ means less than or equal to). For example, if $x_1 = 3$, $x_2 = 5$, $x_3 = 1$ then

$$x_{(1)} = x_3 = 1, \qquad x_{(2)} = x_1 = 3, \qquad x_{(3)} = x_2 = 5.$$

Notation for a population and a sample

A clear distinction must be drawn between the sample and the population from which it was taken. The notation which exemplifies this difference uses Roman letters for the sample statistics and Greek letters for the population parameters which they estimate. Common examples are shown in Table 1.1.

Table 1.1 Notation for a population and a sample

Statistic/parameter	Sample	Population
Mean	$\bar{x}$	μ (mu)
Standard deviation	s	σ (sigma)
Correlation coefficient	r	ρ (rho)
Proportion	p	π (pi)

Examples

Notation

Suppose

$$x_1 = 3, \quad x_2 = 5, \quad x_3 = 1, \quad n = 3$$
$$y_1 = 4, \quad y_2 = 2, \quad y_3 = 10.$$

1. $\displaystyle\sum_{i=1}^{3} x_i y_i = (3)(4)+(5)(2)+(1)(10)$

$$= 12+10+10$$
$$= 32.$$

2. $\displaystyle\sum_{i=1}^{3} (x_i+y_i) = (3+4)+(5+2)+(1+10)$

$$= 7+7+11$$
$$= 25.$$

3. $\displaystyle\sum_{i=1}^{3} 6x_i = 6\sum_{i=1}^{3} x_i$

$$= 6(3+5+1)$$
$$= 54.$$

4. $\displaystyle\sum_{i=1}^{3} 6 = 3(6)$

$$= 18.$$

5. $\displaystyle\prod_{i=1}^{3} x_i = (3)(5)(1) = 15.$

Chapter 2
Descriptive Statistics

Introduction

Descriptive statistics serve as devices for organising data. They may be: (i) tabular; (ii) diagrammatic; or (iii) numerical.

Tables

The tables described relate to a single variable. The concepts may be extended to the consideration of two or more variables.

List

This is the simplest form of a table consisting of two columns, the first giving an identification of the observational unit and the second giving the value of the variable for that unit.

Frequency table

Ungrouped data

A list may be summarised in the form of a frequency table. The first column of this table catalogues all values of the variable (qualitative or quantitative), ordered if feasible, and the second column indicates the corresponding *frequency* of occurrence (i.e. the number of repetitions, the count) of each value. The frequencies are most easily obtained by tallying. Such a table is a *frequency distribution*. This is a technique for systematically arranging a collection of individuals to indicate the frequency of occurrence of the different values of the variable. A frequency distribution may be represented as a table or a histogram (defined below).

Grouped data

When the variable is continuous, it can assume an infinite set of values over a specified range. Thus it is unlikely that many values

will be repeated often. Hence a frequency table of the raw data
will have a negligible advantage over the original listing as an
organisational device, as it is unlikely to differ from it to any great
extent. This holds, too, when the range of values of a discrete
variable is large. In such situations, a summary frequency table is
produced by distributing the data into *classes* or *categories* and
determining the number of individuals belonging to each class, i.e.
the *class frequency*. Data organised and summarised in this way
are called *grouped data*.

General rules for forming a frequency distribution of *grouped
data*:
1. Determine the range of values, R, i.e. the difference between
the largest and smallest values.
2. Decide on the number, I, of classes, also called *class intervals*.
The choice of I is arbitrary. I usually lies between 5 and 20, its
selection depending on the form of the data and the requirements
of the frequency distribution.
3. Determine the width of the class intervals, $w \simeq R/I$. It is convenient to maintain a constant width for all intervals.
4. Choose the upper and the lower limits of the class intervals
such that there are I intervals each of width w and such that each
observation lies strictly *within* a class interval, never on the
boundary between two intervals, so that ambiguities are avoided.
5. List the intervals in order. Consider each observation in turn
and allocate it to the interval into which it falls. Indicate with a
tally. Add the tally marks in each interval to obtain the class
frequencies.

Relative frequency table

Each class (i.e. an interval for grouped data or an observed value
for ungrouped data) contains a proportion of the total frequency.
The proportion for a given class is obtained by dividing the class
frequency by the total frequency for all classes. This proportion is
called the *relative frequency* and is usually expressed as a percentage. The sum of the relative frequencies of all classes is then 100%
(apart from rounding errors). If the frequencies in a frequency
distribution are replaced by relative frequencies, the resulting
distribution is called a *relative frequency distribution*.

Cumulative (relative) frequency table

The cumulative (relative) frequency at a value is the sum of the (relative) frequencies of values less than or equal to that value. When the data are grouped, the value corresponds to the upper limit of the interval concerned.

Diagrams

The form of the diagram varies according to the nature of the data.

Categorical data

Bar chart

This is a graphical representation of (relative) frequencies or magnitudes by rectangles of constant width drawn with lengths proportional to the (relative) frequencies or magnitudes concerned. A bar chart may be: (i) a subdivision of a single bar to indicate the composition of a total; (ii) a comparison of two or more groups utilising bars of varying colours or shades; or (iii) an indication of increase or decrease using bars drawn in opposite directions above and below a zero line.

Pie diagram (circular diagram or chart)

A pie diagram consists of a circle whose area represents the total frequency and which is divided into segments which represent the proportional composition of the total frequency.

Pictogram

This is a diagrammatic representation of (relative) frequencies or magnitudes using symbols (e.g. drawings or pictures) relevant to the subject matter. Symbols of different sizes should not be used, for interpretation then relies on the comparison of areas (which is not easy) rather than lengths, and facts are easily distorted. Instead, a unit value of the data should be represented by a standard symbol which may be repeated to depict magnitude.

Numerical data

One dimensional dot diagram

This is a diagrammatic representation of the distribution of a variable in which every observation is marked as a dot corresponding to its value on a (generally horizontal) line calibrated within the range of values of the variable (e.g. Fig. E2.5).

Scatter diagram (dot graph)

This is a diagrammatic representation of data in a rectangular coordinate system, each observation being represented by a point corresponding to its value on each axis. The value on the horizontal axis is called the *abscissa*; on the vertical axis, the *ordinate*.

Line (polygonal) graph

This is a dot diagram in which successive points relative to the horizontal axis are linked by straight lines. It is appropriate only when the variable on the horizontal axis is continuous and there is at most a single value on the vertical axis corresponding to any value on the horizontal axis. The line graph is called a (cumulative/relative) *frequency polygon* if one axis, commonly the vertical, represents (cumulative/relative) frequency and a *time series* if one axis, commonly the horizontal, represents time. A cumulative frequency polygon is called an *ogive*. A cumulative relative frequency polygon is called a *percentage ogive*.

Histogram

This is a graphical representation of a frequency distribution in which rectangles proportional in *area* to the class frequencies are erected on the horizontal axis, the width of each rectangle corresponding to the class interval of the variable. If the class intervals are of equal size, the heights of the rectangles are proportional, and generally taken to be equal, to the class frequencies. If the class intervals differ in size, the heights must be adjusted accordingly. If the variable is discrete and ungrouped, the rectangles may be replaced by vertical lines. A frequency polygon may be derived from a histogram by connecting the midpoints of the tops of the rectangles in the histogram.

Numerical measures

Two features of the data which characterise a distribution are measures of:

1. Location—central or noncentral.
2. Dispersion (variation, spread, scatter).

The measures are described for ungrouped data for the n observations, $x_1, x_2, \ldots, x_n$. The formulae may be modified for grouped data. Since, in reality, it is virtually impossible in any circumstances to observe all the individuals in a population, for practical purposes, the n observations, $x_1, x_2, \ldots, x_n$, refer to a *sample* of observations.

Measures of location

Common measures of central tendency

In the broadest sense, an *average* is a general term used to describe a value of a variable which is typical or representative of the data. Common types of average are:

1. *Arithmetic mean* ($\bar{x}$)
This is the sum of all the observations divided by the number of observations. It is commonly denoted by $\bar{x}$ (x bar).

$$\bar{x} = \frac{x_1 + x_2 + \ldots + x_n}{n} = \frac{1}{n} \sum_{i=1}^{n} x_i.$$

It is sometimes simply called the mean or the average.

2. *Median*
The middle observation in a set of observations arranged in order of magnitude is known as the median. If $x_{(i)}$ is the value of the variable of rank number i in the ordered series, then for: (i) n *odd*, median = middle value, $x_{([n+1]/2)}$; (ii) n *even*, median = arithmetic mean of middle two values, $\frac{1}{2}[x_{(n/2)} + x_{(n/2+1)}]$.

3. *Mode*
This is the most commonly occurring value in a set of values. The

mode does not exist if all values occur with the same frequency. The distribution is *unimodal* if there is one maximum (peak).

CHOICE OF APPROPRIATE MEASURE OF CENTRAL TENDENCY

A *skewed* distribution is one that is asymmetrical. A unimodal frequency distribution is: (i) *left* (*negatively*) *skewed* if it has a longer tail extending towards lower values of the variable; and (ii) *right* (*positively*) *skewed* if it has a longer tail extending towards higher values of the variable.

The choice of the appropriate measure of central tendency is very much dependent on the nature of the variable under study and the requirements of the measure. As a rough guideline, in a reasonably *symmetric* distribution, the mean is preferred to the median or mode as it utilises the most information and is algebraically defined, and thus amenable to mathematical operations. In a *skewed* distribution, the mean is inappropriate as it is unduly weighted by the outlying observations, and the median is generally favoured. It is hard to estimate the mode from grouped data and, in any case, the mode is often misleading.

EMPIRICAL RELATION BETWEEN THE MEAN, MEDIAN AND MODE

For a unimodal frequency distribution which is:

1. *Symmetric,* mean = mode = median.
2. Moderately *skewed*, mean−mode $\simeq$ 3(mean−median).

Other measures of central tendency

4. *Weighted arithmetic mean* $(\bar{x}_w)$
In some situations, not all the observations have equal importance. For example, some observations might be measured more precisely than others. A rational measure gives relatively more weight to the more precise observations. If the values $x_1, x_2, \ldots, x_k$ have associated weights $w_1, w_2, \ldots, w_k$ then

$$\bar{x}_w = \frac{w_1 x_1 + w_2 x_2 + \ldots + w_k x_k}{w_1 + w_2 + \ldots + w_k} = \frac{\sum_{i=1}^{k} w_i x_i}{\sum_{i=1}^{k} w_i}.$$

If a set of n observations consists of k different values, some or all of which are repeated, such that x_i is a value and w_i its frequency of occurrence ($i = 1, 2, \ldots, k$) then $\sum_{i=1}^{k} w_i = n$ and $\bar{x}_w = \bar{x}$.

5. *Geometric mean* ($\bar{x}_g$)
This is the nth root of the product of the values.

$$\bar{x}_g = \sqrt[n]{(x_1)(x_2) \ldots (x_n)} = \sqrt[n]{\prod_{i=1}^{n} x_i}.$$

The geometric mean is the antilogarithm of the arithmetic mean of the logarithmic values.

Other measures of location

Sometimes measures of location other than those of central tendency are required. The *quantiles* are the $(k-1)$ values of the variable which partition the total frequency into k equal parts when the data are arranged in order of magnitude. Thus the rth quantile, Q_r, has $100r/k\%$ of the observations below it and $100[1-(r/k)]\%$ of the observations above it. Common quantiles are shown in Table 2.1.

Table 2.1 Common quantiles for an ordered data set with k equal partitions of the total frequency

k	Quantile name	No. of quantities	Description in ordered set
2	Median	1	50% of observations both above and below median
4	Quartiles	3	25% of observations below 1st, above 3rd and between successive quartiles
5	Quintiles	4	20% of observations below 1st, above 4th and between successive quintiles
10	Deciles	9	10% of observations below 1st, above 9th and between successive deciles
100	Percentiles	99	1% of observations below 1st, above 99th and between successive percentiles

Median = 2nd quartile = 5th decile = 50th percentile.

Opinions vary on how to determine the exact value of a quantile when the quantile does not coincide with an observation in the set but lies between two of the ordered observations. A practice commonly adopted in this situation is to report simply that the value of the quantile lies between the values of the appropriate adjacent observations, without interpolating between these values. Thus the rth quantile which divides the total frequency into k equal parts, and is calculated from a sample of n observations:

1. Is the observation of rank number $[(r/k)n+1/2]$ if $[(r/k)n+1/2]$ is an integer.
2. Lies between the observations with rank numbers adjacent to $[(r/k)n+1/2]$ if $[(r/k)n+1/2]$ is not an integer.

Measures of dispersion

The average value of a set of observations fails to describe the distribution without the accompaniment of some expression of the degree of dispersion (variation, spread, scatter) of the observations about that average. Common measures of dispersion for a set of n values, $x_1, x_2, \ldots , x_n$, are:

1. *Range*
This is the largest minus the smallest value. Range $= x_{(n)} - x_{(1)}$.
   Advantage: It is easily determined.
   Disadvantages: (i) It does not use directly the majority of the observations; (ii) it is dependent on the number of observations. The range may increase as the number of observations in the sample increases. It never decreases; (iii) a single *outlier* (a value in the extreme of the range separated from the majority) yields a sizeable range, so that, as a measure of dispersion, the range is deceptively large relative to the scatter of most of the values.

2. *Interquartile range*
This is the difference between the third and first quartiles. It is the interval which contains the central 50% of the ordered observations with 25% of them both above and below its upper and lower limits, respectively.
   Advantages: (i) It is unaffected by outliers; (ii) it is independent of the number of observations, i.e. an increase in the number of observations in the sample does not imply an increase in the interquartile range.

Disadvantages: (i) It does not directly use the majority of the observations; (ii) it is clumsy; (iii) it cannot be determined when the number of observations is very small.

Ranges can be determined between any of the quantiles; e.g. *interdecile range* which contains the central 80% of the ordered observations.

Measures exist which directly use all the observations. They quantify the dispersion about a central value by considering the deviation of each observation from the central value. The central value commonly employed is the arithmetic mean, $\bar{x}$. The deviation for the ith observation is $D_i = x_i - \bar{x}$. The arithmetic mean of these deviations is zero:

$$\bar{D} = \frac{\sum D_i}{n} = \frac{\sum (x_i - \bar{x})}{n} = \frac{\sum x_i}{n} - \bar{x} = 0.$$

Therefore measures are devised which overcome the nullifying effect of the opposing signs by utilising either: (i) the *absolute deviation*, $|D_i|$; the sign of the deviation is ignored and every deviation is considered positive; or (ii) the *square of the deviation*, D_i^2, a positive quantity (see Fig. 2.1).

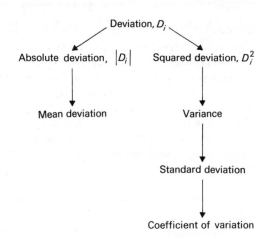

Fig. 2.1 Measures of dispersion using D_i.

3. *Mean deviation*
If the population of observations is available, the mean deviation is the *arithmetic mean of the absolute deviations*, i.e. $\sum^{N} |x_i - \mu|/N$, where N is the number of observations in the popu-

lation, and μ is the population mean. As noted previously, in practice one is generally forced to consider only a sample of observations which can provide only an estimate of the true mean deviation. It can be shown that for a sample of n observations, a very good estimator of the mean deviation of the population from which the sample is taken is

$$\frac{1}{n-1} \sum_{i}^{n} |x_i - \bar{x}|.$$

Advantage: It uses every observation.
Disadvantage: It is difficult to manipulate mathematically.

4. *Variance, Var (x)*
If the population of observations is available, the variance is the *arithmetic mean of the squared deviations*, i.e.

$$\sigma^2 = \sum^{N} (x_i - \mu)^2 / N.$$

where N is the number of observations in the population, and μ is the population mean. In practice, generally one considers only a sample of observations and a very good estimator of the variance of the population derived from a sample of n observations can be shown to be

$$s^2 = \frac{\sum^{n}(x_i - \bar{x})^2}{n-1}.$$

The numerator, $\sum(x_i - \bar{x})^2$, is called the *sum of squares about the mean* or the *corrected sum of squares*. The estimated variance is most easily calculated using the equivalent formula:

$$s^2 = \frac{1}{n-1} \left[\sum x_i^2 - \frac{(\sum x_i)^2}{n} \right].$$

Advantages: (i) It uses every observation; (ii) it is mathematically manageable.
Disadvantage: Its dimensionality is that of the square of the original observations.

5. *Standard deviation, SD (x)*
The standard deviation is the positive square root of the variance.

The sample estimator of the population standard deviation is

$$s = \sqrt{\frac{1}{n-1} \sum (x_i - \bar{x})^2} = \sqrt{\frac{1}{n-1}\left(\sum x_i^2 - \frac{(\sum x_i)^2}{n}\right)}.$$

Advantages: (i) It uses every observation; (ii) it is mathematically manageable; (iii) its dimensionality is that of the original observations.

Disadvantage: It is very sensitive to outliers.

The *intuitive appeal* of the standard deviation as an indicator of the dispersion of the observations is apparent when it is considered:

a. In the context of a normal distribution (see Chapter 4). For example, if the observations are normally distributed, approximately 95% of them are contained in the interval which spans the mean by two standard deviations on either side of it.

b. As a sort of average deviation about the mean. Some deviations are greater than the standard deviation and some deviations are less than the standard deviation.

Coefficient of variation, *CV* (x)

The interpretation of an absolute measure of dispersion depends on the scale of the observations. The effect of the magnitude of the observations is removed by *standardising* the absolute measure of dispersion by a quantity which is representative of the magnitude, i.e. an average. In general terms:

$$\text{Relative measure of dispersion} = \frac{\text{Absolute measure of dispersion}}{\text{Average}}.$$

In particular, when the absolute measure of dispersion is the standard deviation and the average is the arithmetic mean, the quotient is called the *coefficient of variation*. It is generally expressed as a percentage. In symbols, the coefficient of variation estimated from a sample of observations is:

$$CV(x) = \frac{s}{\bar{x}} \, 100\%.$$

Advantage: It is dimensionless, independent of units used.

Disadvantages: (i) It may be misleading in the absence of specific knowledge of the mean and standard deviation; (ii) it is statistically awkward; (iii) it can only be used when $\bar{x} > 0$.

Examples

Tables

Table E2.1 Skinfold thicknesses (mm) measured at the triceps mid-point of 55 male subjects

18.4	11.4	14.3	12.6	9.4	11.1	20.4	15.7	17.6	14.8	10.7
15.3	11.7	13.9	18.9	9.6	7.9	23.7	21.3	17.3	16.8	7.9
9.1	11.4	16.8	10.7	15.1	16.6	13.3	16.2	9.5	11.3	7.6
18.4	12.7	11.4	14.8	13.6	18.5	4.9	14.9	13.6	11.3	23.3
10.9	18.2	27.3	17.8	13.6	16.2	8.3	9.9	12.4	11.4	9.6

Source: Hypothetical data.

Table E2.2 (Frequency/rel. freq./cum. freq./cum. rel. freq. table)

Skinfold thickness (mm)	Tally	Frequency	Relative frequency (%)	Cumulative frequency	Cum. rel. frequency (%)
0.0–	I	1	1.8	1	1.8
5.0–	ЖН ЖН	10	18.2	11	20.0
10.0–	ЖН ЖН ЖН ЖН III	23	41.8	34	61.8
15.0–	ЖН ЖН ЖН I	16	29.0	50	90.8
20.0–	IIII	4	7.2	54	98.0
25.0–29.9	I	1	1.8	55	99.8
Total		55	99.8		

Source: Table E2.1.

Diagrams

The data of Table E2.3 are used to illustrate the diagrammatic forms discussed in Chapter 2.

Table E2.3 Legitimate total births, England and Wales, 1969–70

	Mother's age (years)		
Parity	< 30	≥ 30	Total (all ages)
0	514 108	49 895	564 003
1–3	583 889	234 084	817 973
≥ 4	22 216	64 894	87 110
Total (all parities)	1 120 213	348 873	1 469 086

Source: Osborn, J.F. (1975) *J.R. Statist. Soc.* (C), **24**, 75–84.

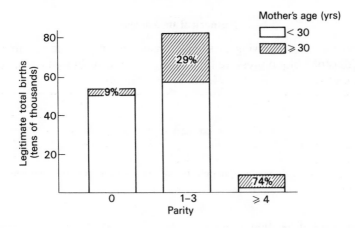

Fig. E2.1 Bar chart. Source: Table E2.3.

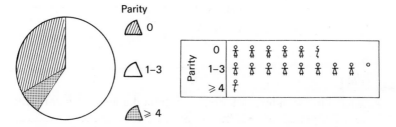

Fig. E2.2 (*left*) Pie diagram. Proportional composition of mothers (all ages) by parity. Source: Table E2.3.

Fig. E2.3 (*right*) Pictogram. Numbers of mothers (all ages) in hundreds of thousands. Source: Table E2.3.

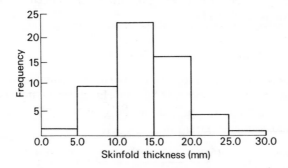

Fig. E2.4 Histogram. Distribution of skinfold thickness. Source: Table E2.2.

Numerical measures

Consider the following 11 sample measurements of the variable, x [diastolic blood pressure (mm Hg)], whose distribution is shown in Fig. E2.5: 71, 81, 85, 94, 88, 84, 82, 86, 86, 79, 77.

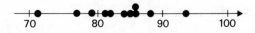

Fig. E2.5 Distribution of diastolic blood pressure measurements (mm Hg).

Measures of location

Arithmetic mean

$$\bar{x} = (71+81+\ldots+77)/11$$
$$= (913)/11$$
$$= 83 \text{ mm Hg.}$$

Median

Arranged in ascending order of magnitude the measurements are: 71, 77, 79, 81, 82, 84, 85, 86, 86, 88, 94.

$$x_{([n+1]/2)} = x_{([11+1]/2)} = x_{(6)} = 84 \text{ mm Hg.}$$

Mode

The value 86 occurs twice whilst all other values occur only once. The mode is 86 mm Hg.

Weighted arithmetic mean

If consideration is given to another five measurements of diastolic BP whose arithmetic mean is 89 mm Hg, the weighted mean of the two arithmetic means, taking the weights as the number of observations in each group, is

$$\bar{x}_w = \frac{(5)(89)+(11)(83)}{5+11} = 84.9 \text{ mm Hg.}$$

Geometric mean

$$\overline{x}_g = \sqrt[11]{(71)(81)\ldots(77)}$$
$$= \sqrt[11]{1.25 \times 10^{21}}$$
$$= 82.8 \text{ mm Hg.}$$

Quantiles

25th percentile $=$ 1st quartile
$$= x_{([11+1]/4)} = x_{(3)} = 79 \text{ mm Hg.}$$
75th percentile $=$ 3rd quartile
$$= x_{([11+1]3/4)} = x_{(9)} = 86 \text{ mm Hg.}$$

Measures of dispersion

Range

$$94-71 = 23 \text{ mm Hg.}$$

Interquartile range

3rd quartile$-$1st quartile $= 86-79 = 7$ mm Hg.

Estimated mean deviation

$$\frac{\sum |x_i - \overline{x}|}{n-1} = \frac{50}{11} = 4.6 \text{ mm Hg (see Table E2.4).}$$

Estimated variance

$$s^2 = \frac{\sum (x_i - \overline{x})^2}{n-1} = \frac{370}{10} = 37 \text{ mm}^2 \text{ Hg}$$

or

$$s^2 = \frac{\sum x_i^2 - (\sum x_i)^2/n}{n-1} = \frac{1}{10} [76149 - (913)^2/11]$$

$$= \frac{1}{10} (76149 - 75779)$$

$$= 370/10$$

$$= 37 \text{ mm}^2 \text{ Hg}$$

(See Table E2.4.)

Chapter 2

Table E2.4 Calculations for the estimation of the mean deviation and variance

	x_i	$x_i - \bar{x}^*$	$|x_i - \bar{x}|$	x_i^2	$(x_i - \bar{x})^2$
	71	-12	12	5041	144
	81	-2	2	6561	4
	85	2	2	7225	4
	94	11	11	8836	121
	88	5	5	7744	25
	84	1	1	7056	1
	82	-1	1	6724	1
	86	3	3	7396	9
	86	3	3	7396	9
	79	-4	4	6241	16
	77	-6	6	5929	36
Total	913	0	50	76149	370

$^*\bar{x} = 83$.
Source: 11 measurements of diastolic BP (mm Hg).

Estimated standard deviation

$$s = \sqrt{37} = 6.1 \text{ mm Hg.}$$

Estimated coefficient of variation

$$\text{CV}(x) = \frac{s}{\bar{x}} \, 100 = \left(\frac{6.1}{83}\right) 100 = 7.3\%.$$

Chapter 3
Probability

Introduction

Inferential statistics is concerned with drawing conclusions about a population on the basis of the information assimilated from a sample drawn from the population. An element of uncertainty is associated with every conclusion, a consequence of the non-totality of the information. This uncertainty is formally and numerically expressed as a *probability*. The theory of probability is the foundation of statistical inference.

Definition of probability

Probability may be viewed in various ways, most commonly as subjective probability, *a priori* probability and empirical probability.

Subjective probability

Subjective probability is personalistic and thus indefinable, expressing the *degrees of belief* that a person holds for different eventualities (e.g. the probability that a cure for cancer will be found within the next 5 years). Subjective probability is determined by an individual on the basis of the relevant personal experience he brings to bear on the situation. Subjective probability may vary from one person to another in that their experience and ways of viewing experience may be different.

A priori probability

Suppose there are n equally likely outcomes to a trial, and an event, E, consists of n_E of these outcomes. Then the probability of occurrence of E (called its *success,* denoted by E) is

$$p = \Pr(E) = \frac{n_E}{n}.$$

25

The probability of non-occurrence of E (its *failure*, denoted by $\overline{E}$) is

$$q = \text{Pr}\,(\overline{E}) = \frac{n - n_E}{n} = 1 - p.$$

Such probabilities form the basis of much of genetics.

Empirical probability

If a procedure is repeated many times, the proportion of times the event occurs out of the total number of repetitions is approximately equal to the *a priori* probability. Exact equality is achieved for an infinite number of repetitions. Thus the probability of an event pertaining to a procedure may be defined as the *relative frequency* of occurrence of the event in a very large number of repetitions of the procedure.

Explanation of terms

The terms are considered for two events. The concepts may be extended for more than two events.

Independence

Two events are *independent* if the occurrence or non-occurrence (the outcome) of one event does not affect the probability of the outcome of the other. Otherwise they are *dependent* events.

Mutual exclusiveness

Two events are mutually exclusive if the occurrence of one of them excludes the occurrence of the other.

Conditional probability

If the probability of the outcome of one event, E_1, *is* affected by the outcome of the second event, E_2, then the probability of E_1 is said to be *conditional* on E_2. The conditional probability of E_1, *given* that E_2 has occurred, is written $\text{Pr}(E_1 | E_2)$.

Properties of probabilities

1. $0 \le \Pr(E) \le 1$ for any event E.
In particular if:

    a. $\Pr(E) = 0$, the event, E, *cannot* occur.
    b. $\Pr(E) = 1$, the event, E, *must* occur.

2. The sum of the probabilities attached to all mutually exclusive outcomes of a procedure is unity. Thus if a procedure has k mutually exclusive outcomes, $E_1, E_2, \ldots, E_k$, with respective probabilities $\Pr(E_1), \Pr(E_2), \ldots, \Pr(E_k)$, then

$$\sum_{i=1}^{k} \Pr(E_i) = 1.$$

Useful formulae

The formulae relate to two events, E_1 and E_2. They may be extended for more than two events. The formulae centre on the two conjunctions *and* and *or*. Expressions are given for the probability of occurrence of: (i) E_1 *and* E_2, written $\Pr(E_1E_2)$; (ii) E_1 *or* E_2, written $\Pr(E_1+E_2)$ in different circumstances.

Multiplication rule

$$\mathbf{Pr}(E_1E_2)$$

Events independent

If E_1 and E_2 are independent of each other, then the probability of both E_1 *and* E_2 occurring is the *product* of the probability of each.

$$\Pr(E_1E_2) = \Pr(E_1)\Pr(E_2). \tag{3.1}$$

Events not necessarily independent

$$\Pr(E_1E_2) = \Pr(E_2)\Pr(E_1|E_2) = \Pr(E_1)\Pr(E_2|E_1). \tag{3.2}$$

Equation (3.2) reduces to equation (3.1) when E_1 and E_2 *are* independent for then $\Pr(E_2|E_1) = \Pr(E_2)$ and $\Pr(E_1|E_2) = \Pr(E_1)$.

Chapter 3

Addition rule

$$\mathbf{Pr}(E_1+E_2)$$

Events mutually exclusive

The probability of either E_1 *or* E_2 occurring, if they are mutually exclusive, is equal to the *sum* of the probability of each.

$$\Pr(E_1+E_2) = \Pr(E_1)+\Pr(E_2). \tag{3.3}$$

Events not necessarily mutually exclusive

The probability of either E_1 *or* E_2 *or both* E_1 and E_2 occurring (i.e. E_1 and E_2 are not necessarily mutually exclusive) is

$$\Pr(E_1+E_2) = \Pr(E_1)+\Pr(E_2)-\Pr(E_1E_2). \tag{3.4}$$

Equation (3.4) reduces to equation (3.3) when E_1 and E_2 *are* mutually exclusive for then $\Pr(E_1E_2) = 0$.

Examples

A priori probability

Suppose a trial consists of drawing a card at random from a deck of 52 cards. Every card has an equal chance of being selected (an outcome $\equiv$ a selected card). Let the event, E, be that an Ace is drawn. The probability of drawing an Ace is the ratio of the number of Aces in the deck (the number of successful outcomes) to the number of cards in the deck (the total number of possible outcomes), i.e. $\Pr(\text{Ace}) = 4/52 = 1/13$.

Empirical probability

Suppose a trial consists of drawing a card at random from a deck of 52 cards. Every card has an equal chance of being selected. Suppose also that the trial is repeated 1000 times, the selected card being replaced in the deck at the end of each trial. The empirical probability of an Ace being drawn is the ratio of the actual number of Aces drawn to the number of trials performed. Thus if 70 Aces are drawn in 1000 trials, the empirical probability of an Ace drawn is $70/1000 = 0.070$. This is approximately equal to $1/13 = 0.077$, the *a priori* probability.

Explanation of terms

Independence

Consider a deck of 52 cards from which two cards are drawn at random, the first card being replaced in the deck after its selection. The probability of an Ace being selected in the second draw is 1/13, whether an Ace was drawn initially or not. The selection of an Ace in the second draw is independent of the selection of an Ace in the first draw.

Mutual exclusiveness

Consider a deck of 52 cards from which a single card is drawn at random. If the card drawn is an Ace, then clearly that card cannot be a King. The two events (drawing an Ace and drawing a King) are mutually exclusive.

Conditional probability

Consider a deck of 52 cards from which two cards are drawn at random and the first card is not replaced in the deck after its selection. The probability of selecting an Ace as the second card is dependent on what was drawn as the first card. For example, if the card drawn first was an Ace ($\Pr(\text{Ace}) = 4/52$) then the second card is selected from the remaining 51 cards in which there are only three Aces. The probability of the second card being an Ace is thus 3/51. This latter probability is the conditional probability of selecting an Ace as the second card given that an Ace was selected initially.

Useful formulae

Consider a deck of 52 cards. When a selection is made from the deck, each card has an equal chance of being chosen.

Multiplication rule

1. *Events independent:* Two cards are selected from the deck, the first card being replaced after its selection.

$$E_1 = \text{Ace in first draw}, \Pr(E_1) = 4/52 = 0.077$$
$$E_2 = \text{Ace in second draw}, \Pr(E_2) = 4/52 = 0.077.$$

E_1 and E_2 are independent events. The probability of both cards drawn being Aces is

$$\Pr(E_1E_2) = \Pr(E_1)\Pr(E_2) = (4/52)(4/52) = 0.006.$$

2. *Events not necessarily independent:* Two cards are selected from the deck, the first card not being replaced after its selection.

E_1 = Ace in first draw, $\Pr(E_1) = 4/52 = 0.077$
E_2 = Ace in second draw, $\Pr(E_2|E_1) = 3/51 = 0.059$.

E_1 and E_2 are dependent events. The probability of both cards drawn being aces is

$$\begin{aligned}\Pr(E_1E_2) &= \Pr(E_1)\Pr(E_2|E_1)\\&= (4/52)(3/51) = 0.005.\end{aligned}$$

Additional rule

1. *Events mutually exclusive:* One card is selected from the deck.

E_1 = Ace is drawn, $\Pr(E_1) = 4/52 = 0.077$
E_2 = King is drawn, $\Pr(E_2) = 4/52 = 0.077$.

E_1 and E_2 are mutually exclusive. The probability of drawing either an Ace or a King is

$$\begin{aligned}\Pr(E_1+E_2) &= \Pr(E_1)+\Pr(E_2)\\&= (4/52)+(4/52) = 0.154.\end{aligned}$$

2. *Events not necessarily mutually exclusive:* One card is selected from the deck.

E_1 = Ace is drawn, $\Pr(E_1) = 4/52 = 0.077$
E_2 = Heart is drawn, $\Pr(E_2) = 13/52 = 0.25$.

E_1 and E_2 are not mutually exclusive. The probability of drawing an Ace or a Heart or the Ace of Hearts is

$$\begin{aligned}\Pr(E_1+E_2) &= \Pr(E_1)+\Pr(E_2)-\Pr(E_1E_2)\\&= (4/52)+(13/52)-(1/52)\\&= 0.308.\end{aligned}$$

Chapter 4
Probability Distributions

Definition

Inferences are made about a population by constructing a formal *model* of the situation. This model consists of a statement of the possible outcomes relative to the situation and an assumption about their respective probabilities. A *complete* statement of this form defines a *probability distribution*. Formally:

A *random variable* is a quantity which takes any of the values of a specified set with a specified probability.

The (probability) *distribution* of a random variable is a table, graph or mathematical expression giving the probabilities with which the random variable takes different values.

Mean and variance of a probability distribution

The mean and variance of a probability distribution may be defined in terms of *expectation*.

For a *discrete* random variable, x, taking the values $x_1, x_2, \ldots, x_k$ with respective probabilities $p_1, p_2, \ldots, p_k$, where $\sum_{i=1}^{k} p_i = 1$, the *expectation* (expected value) of x is

$$E(x) = \sum_{i=1}^{k} p_i x_i.$$

The expectation of a *continuous* random variable may be defined analogously, but the definition involves a mathematical technique, more complex than summation, called integration.

In either case, for the random variable x:

1. $E(x) = \mu$, the mean of the probability distribution of x.
2. $E(x-\mu)^2 = \sigma^2$, the variance of the probability distribution of x.

Probability distributions may be: (i) discrete; or (ii) continuous; depending on whether the random variable of interest is discrete or continuous.

31

Discrete probability distributions

A *discrete probability distribution* is one in which the random variable, x, takes the discrete values $x_1, x_2, \ldots, x_k$ with respective probabilities $p_1, p_2, \ldots, p_k$ such that the sum of all the probabilities is unity, i.e.

$$\sum_{i=1}^{k} p_i = 1.$$

A discrete probability distribution is analogous to a relative frequency distribution with probabilities replacing relative frequencies. It may be presented diagrammatically in the form of a histogram with rectangles proportional in area to probabilities.

The *probability function* or *frequency function* of x, $p(x)$, is the mathematical expression which assumes the values $p_1, p_2, \ldots, p_k$ for $x = x_1, x_2, \ldots, x_k$.

Common discrete probability distributions are the: (i) binomial; and (ii) Poisson.

Binomial distribution

The binomial distribution is relevant in cases where there are two outcomes to a trial, success (with probability π) or failure (with probability $1-\pi$) and the trial is repeated n times, each repetition being independent. The random variable of interest, x, is the number of successes in the n trials. The binomial distribution is the probability distribution of x. For a particular value of x equal to r ($r = 0, 1, 2, \ldots, n$), it determines the probability of observing exactly r successes in the n trials. These probabilities may be evaluated from:

1. First principles, using the probability formulae expressed in Chapter 3.
2. The probability function

$$\Pr(x = r) = \frac{n!}{(n-r)!r!}\, \pi^r (1-\pi)^{n-r},$$

where $n!$ (n factorial) is $n! = n(n-1)(n-2) \ldots (3)(2)(1); 0! = 1$, by definition.

π may be known *a priori* or it may be estimated empirically as

$p = r/n$, the ratio of the number of successes observed in the n trials to the number of trials.

Properties of the binomial distribution

1. Characterised by n and π.
2. Mean $= n\pi$.
3. Variance $= n\pi(1-\pi)$.
4. Standard deviation $= \sqrt{n\pi(1-\pi)}$.

Poisson distribution

The Poisson distribution is the probability distribution of the number of events, x, which occur independently and randomly in:

1. Time, at a fixed rate per unit time, such that the probability of occurrence of more than one event in a short interval of time is very small as compared to the length of the interval.
2. Space, with a fixed density per unit area (volume), such that the probability of occurrence of more than one event in a small area (volume) is very small as compared to the size of area (volume).

The probability of r events occurring is

$$\Pr(x = r) = \frac{\exp(-\mu)\mu^r}{r!} \text{ for } r = 0, 1, 2, \ldots,$$

where $e = 2.718$ is the base of natural (Naperian) logarithms and $\exp(-\mu)$ is the exponential function $e^{-\mu}$; $r! = (r)(r-1)(r-2) \ldots (3)(2)(1)$.

μ may be known *a priori* or it may be estimated from the sample by $\bar{x}$, the arithmetic mean.

Properties of the Poisson distribution

1. Characterised by μ.
2. Mean $= \mu$.
3. Variance $= \mu$.
4. Standard deviation $= \sqrt{\mu}$.
5. The Poisson distribution approximates the binomial distribution when the number of trials, n, is large and the probability of success in a single trial, π, is small. For if π is small, $1-\pi \simeq 1$ and the variance of the binomial distribution is approximately equal to $n\pi$ which is the mean of the binomial distribution.

Continuous probability distributions

The concepts of a discrete probability distribution may be extended to the situation in which the random variable of interest, x, is continuous and can thus assume an infinite set of values over a specified range (see Table 4.1).

Table 4.1 Analogues of $p(x)$ for the random variable, x

		$p(x)$	
x	Nomenclature	Interpretation	Diagrammatic representation
Discrete	Probability (frequency) function	Probability	Probability histogram
Continuous	Probability density function	Probability density	Continuous curve

1. The *total area* under the probability density function, $p(x)$, bounded by the x axis is unity. This corresponds to the sum, equal to one, of the probabilities associated with all values of a discrete random variable.

2. The *partial area* under the probability density function, $p(x)$, bounded by the x axis and any two lines $x = a$ and $x = b$, is equivalent to the probability that x lies between the values a and b, $\Pr(a < x < b)$. This is the shaded area in Fig. 4.1 and is evaluated by a mathematical technique called integration.

The most common *examples* of continuous probability distributions are the normal, t, χ^2 and F distributions. The normal distribution is discussed below. The other continuous distributions are discussed in Chapter 5.

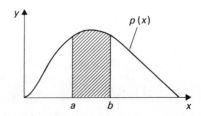

Fig. 4.1 Probability density function, $p(x)$, of a continuous random variable, x.

Normal (Gaussian) distribution

The probability density function of the normal distribution is

$$p(x) = \frac{1}{\sqrt{(2\pi)}\sigma} \exp[-(x-\mu)^2/(2\sigma^2)] \qquad (-\infty < x < \infty) \quad (4.1)$$

Properties of the normal distribution

1. Characterised by two parameters, μ and σ^2. The notation $N(\mu, \sigma^2)$ thus fully describes the distribution.
2. Mean $= \mu$.
3. Variance $= \sigma^2$.
4. Standard deviation $= \sigma$.
5. Unimodal.
6. Symmetric about μ.
7. A change in μ from μ_1 to μ_2 (for constant σ) shifts the curve along the x axis to the right (if $\mu_2 > \mu_1$) or to the left (if $\mu_2 < \mu_1$).
8. A change in σ from σ_1 to σ_2 (for constant μ) alters the peakedness of the curve so that it is more peaked (if $\sigma_1 > \sigma_2$) or less peaked (if $\sigma_1 < \sigma_2$): i.e. decreasing σ, a measure of dispersion, makes the distribution tall and thin; increasing σ makes the distribution fat and flat.
9. The intervals spanning the mean, μ, by σ, 2σ and 3σ on either side of μ enclose respectively 68.27%, 95.45% and 99.73% of the total probability. Thus:

$$\Pr(\mu-\sigma < x < \mu+\sigma) \simeq 0.68$$
$$\Pr(\mu-2\sigma < x < \mu+2\sigma) \simeq 0.95$$
$$\Pr(\mu-3\sigma < x < \mu+3\sigma) \simeq 1.$$

In fact,

$$\Pr(\mu-1.96\sigma < x < \mu+1.96\sigma) = 0.95.$$

Standard normal distribution

If the random variable x is normally distributed with mean μ and variance σ^2 [written x dist. $N(\mu, \sigma^2)$], then the probability that x lies between any two values a and b is equal to the area under the probability density function $p(x)$ given in equation (4.1), between the x axis and the boundaries $x = a$ and $x = b$. This area may be determined by the mathematical integration of $p(x)$ evaluated between the limits $x = a$ and $x = b$. Since the integration is too complex to be practically viable for all combinations of a and b, simplification of method is necessary. This is achieved by performing the integration only once for a particular normal distribution, the *standard normal distribution, N*(0, 1), with zero mean and unit variance. The results are expressed as probabilities and are tabulated (Table A1).

Any normally distributed random variable x may be transformed to a variable $z = (x-\mu)/\sigma$ having a standard normal distribution. The probability that x lies between a and b is then equivalent to the probability that $z = (x-\mu)/\sigma$ lies between $(a-\mu)/\sigma$ and $(b-\mu)/\sigma$ and is tabulated. z is called the *standard normal deviate,* SND. The probability density function for the standard normal deviate, z, is

$$p(z) = \frac{1}{\sqrt{(2\pi)}} \exp(-\tfrac{1}{2}z^2) \qquad (-\infty < z < +\infty)$$

Tables of the standard normal distribution

The areas under the standard normal distribution may be tabulated as probabilities in different ways, as shown in Fig. 4.2.

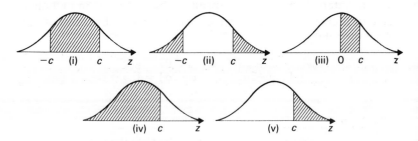

Fig. 4.2 Tabulated integrals (probabilities) of the standard normal distribution with probability density function $p(z)$.

The shaded area under each curve in Fig. 4.2 corresponds to the tabulated probability associated with a value, c, of z. Any one of these tabulations may be used to obtain the probability of interest if it is remembered that: (i) $p(z)$ is symmetrical about $z = 0$; (ii) the total area between $p(z)$ and the z axis is unity. Then:

1. $\Pr(z < -c) = \Pr(z > c)$.
2. $\Pr(z > c) = 1 - \Pr(z < c)$.
3. $\Pr(z > -c) = 1 - \Pr(z > c)$.
4. $\Pr(a < z < b) = \Pr(z < b) - \Pr(z < a)$ for any two values a, $b(a < b)$.

Table A1 tabulates the probabilities indicated by the shaded area in curve (v) of Fig. 4.2. In it, a percentage point is explicitly related to the probability indicated by the shaded area by using the notation $Z(\alpha)$, instead of c, to describe that value of z beyond which lies $100\alpha\%$ of the total probability.

Approximations by the normal distribution

1. *Binomial*
The normal distribution approximates the binomial distribution as n increases, although less rapidly if π is close to 0 or 1. The approximation is very good if both $n\pi$ and $n(1-\pi)$ are greater than 5. The binomial random variable x, for large enough n, is approximately normally distributed with mean $n\pi$ and variance $n\pi(1-\pi)$. The standard normal deviate of a particular value of x equal to r is

$$z = \frac{r - n\pi}{\sqrt{[n\pi(1-\pi)]}}.$$

2. *Poisson*
The Poisson random variable x, for large enough n, is approximately normally distributed with mean μ. The standard normal deviate of a particular value of x equal to r is $z = (r-\mu)/\sqrt{\mu}$.

Continuity correction

Both the binomial and Poisson distributions are discrete probability distributions whilst the normal distribution is a continuous probability distribution. A *continuity correction* is introduced to allow for the discrepancy if the normal distribution is used to approximate the binomial or Poisson distributions. The continuity correction is the quantity $1/2$ (or $1/(2n)$ in the case of a proportion) which is subtracted from the absolute value of the numerator of the standard normal deviate.

Examples

Discrete probability distributions

Binomial distribution

Suppose a 'trial' consists of investigating the sex of a child at birth, a boy representing a success and a girl representing a failure. The (assumed constant) probability of success (i.e. of a male birth) in the general population is known to be 0.51, i.e. this is the proportion of male births in the population. A particular study is concerned with mothers who bear exactly four children (equivalent to the trial being repeated four times). It is of interest to determine the probability that a mother of this fecundity, selected at random, bears: 0 boys (0 successes, $r = 0$); 1 boy (1 success, $r = 1$); 2 boys; 3 boys; 4 boys. These probabilities are determined from the formula:

$$\Pr(x = r) = \frac{n!}{(n-r)!r!} \, \pi^r (1-\pi)^{n-r} \quad \text{for } r = 0, 1, 2, 3, 4,$$

where x, the random variable of interest, is the number of boys in the four births; $n = 4$; $\pi = 0.51$.

The estimated probabilities are shown in Table E4.1.

Table E4.1 Probabilities of r male births for mothers bearing four children

r	$(n!)/[(n-r)!r!]$	0.51^r	0.49^{4-r}	$P(x = r)$
0	1	1.00	0.058	0.06
1	4	0.51	0.118	0.24
2	6	0.26	0.240	0.37
3	4	0.13	0.490	0.26
4	1	0.07	1.000	0.07
Total				1.00

Thus, for example, the probability of a mother of this fecundity bearing two boys is 0.37.

Note: It may be of interest to determine in advance of selecting a sample of mothers of this fecundity (100 mothers, say) how many of them would be *expected* to bear a specified number of boys (two boys, say). The expected number of mothers bearing two boys in a random sample of 100 mothers each bearing four children is $100\Pr(x = 2) = 100(0.037) = 37$.

Poisson distribution

Table E4.2 shows a distribution observed during a microscopic count of islands in a plane section of the pancreas. The probability of $x = r(r = 0, 1, 2, \ldots, 6)$ islands per square is calculated from the formula $\Pr(x = r) = \exp(-\mu)\mu^r/r!$ where μ is estimated by the sample mean,

$$\bar{x} = [(327)(0) + (340)(1) + \ldots + (1)(6)]/900 = 1.0044$$

(*note:* $\text{Var}(x)$ is calculated to be $1.019 \simeq \bar{x}$). The enumerated probabilities and expected numbers are given in Table E4.3 for $r = 0, 1, 2, \ldots, 6$. The expected number of squares evaluated assuming a Poisson distribution of counts agrees well with those observed for each value of $r(r = 0, 1, \ldots, 6)$.

Table E4.2 Distribution of microscopic counts of islands in a plane section of the pancreas

Number of islands per square (r)	0	1	2	3	4	5	6	Total
Number of squares with r islands	327	340	160	53	16	3	1	900

Source: Hypothetical data.

Table E4.3 Poisson distribution of counts of islands (x) in a plane section of the pancreas

		Number of squares with r islands	
r	$\Pr(x = r)$	Expected $[900\Pr(x = r)]$	Observed
0	$\exp(-\mu) = 0.3662$	329.6	327
1	$\exp(-\mu)(\mu) = 0.3678$	331.0	340
2	$\Pr(x = 1)(\mu/2) = 0.1848$	166.3	160
3	$\Pr(x = 2)(\mu/3) = 0.0619$	55.7	53
4	$\Pr(x = 3)(\mu/4) = 0.0155$	14.0	16
5	$\Pr(x = 4)(\mu/5) = 0.0031$	2.8	3
6	$\Pr(x = 5)(\mu/6) = 0.0005$	0.5	1
Total	1.0000	899.9	900

Source: Table E4.2.

Chapter 5
Sampling and Sampling Distributions

Random sampling

Statistical inference relies on the formal projection of knowledge from the sample to the population. This projection is based on the assumption that the sample is representative of the population from which it is drawn, in the variable(s) under study. Representativeness is ensured by *random sampling,* in which every individual in the population is selected by chance methods. Random number tables are commonly used as the device for selecting the individuals to be included in the random sample, although mechanical methods, such as tossing a coin, are an alternative.

Sampling errors

A consequence of the non-totality of the information contained in a sample is some error in the estimates of the population parameters. This error is called *sampling error.* The sampling error may be controlled by the sample *size* and the sample *design* (method of data collection) used. Retaining the basic attribute of randomness, the best design for a given problem is the one which provides the necessary precision, in terms of the sampling error, for a minimum cost. [*Note: Precision* refers to the way in which repeated observations conform to themselves. *Accuracy* refers to the closeness of an observed value of a quantity (e.g. $\bar{x}$) to its true value (e.g. μ).] Some of the common designs are simple random sampling, stratified random sampling, cluster sampling and systematic sampling.

Sampling distributions

In order to evaluate the sampling error of a sample statistic (e.g. $\bar{x}$) which estimates a population parameter (e.g. μ), the distribution of this statistic (its sampling distribution) must be determined. The sampling distribution of a statistic is the distribution obtained by

40

computing the statistic for all possible samples of a predetermined size which can be drawn from a given population. If there are k possible samples of size n, there will be many ($\leq k$) different values of the statistic. These values form their own distribution, the sampling distribution of the statistic, which has its own mean, variance, etc. The standard deviation of the distribution of a statistic is usually called the *standard error,* and it is this which gives an indication of the adequacy of the statistic as an estimator of the parameter. The distribution of a statistic is essentially a theoretical distribution in that in practice, rarely, if ever, are all possible samples drawn from a population. A large finite population may, for practical purposes, be approximated by an infinite population. The properties of the sampling distributions considered in the text relate to an infinite population. Some adjustments are necessary when the population is finite.

Distribution of the sample mean, $\bar{x}$

The distribution of the sample mean of a variable x is determined by computing the sample means ($\bar{x}_1$, $\bar{x}_2$, . . . , $\bar{x}_k$) for all the k possible samples of size n which can be drawn from the population of values ($x_1, x_2, . . . , x_N$). If the distribution of the observations comprising the parent population has mean μ and variance σ^2, then the distribution of the sample mean has mean $\mu_{\bar{x}}$ and variance $\sigma^2_{\bar{x}}$ such that:

1. Mean, $\mu_{\bar{x}} = \mu$, i.e. $\bar{x}$ is an unbiased estimator of μ. (A statistic is an *unbiased* estimator of a parameter if the mean of the sampling distribution of the statistic is the parameter.)
2. Variance, $\sigma^2_{\bar{x}} = \sigma^2/n$.
3. Standard error of the mean [SEM, SE ($\bar{x}$)], $\sigma_{\bar{x}} = \sigma/\sqrt{n}$.
4. The sampling distribution is approximately *normal* when the distribution of the parent population is: (i) normal (in fact, the sampling distribution *is* normal); (ii) of any form, not necessarily normal, provided n is large ($n \geq 30$, say).

Distributions of the sum of and difference between two independent sample means

The distributions of the sum of and the difference between two independent sample means from two populations may be determined in a similar fashion, by considering the combination of all possible independent samples from the two populations. For the ith population ($i = 1, 2$), the distribution of the sample mean, $\bar{x}_i$, has mean $\mu_{\bar{x}_i}$ and variance $\sigma^2_{\bar{x}_i}$.

Distribution of the sum of two independent sample means, $\bar{x}_1 + \bar{x}_2$

1. Mean, $\mu_{\bar{x}_1 + \bar{x}_2} = \mu_{\bar{x}_1} + \mu_{\bar{x}_2}$.
2. Variance, $\sigma^2_{\bar{x}_1 + \bar{x}_2} = \sigma^2_{\bar{x}_1} + \sigma^2_{\bar{x}_2}$.
3. Standard error, $\sigma_{\bar{x}_1 + \bar{x}_2} = \sqrt{\sigma^2_{\bar{x}_1} + \sigma^2_{\bar{x}_2}}$.
4. The distribution is (approximately) normal if both sampling distributions of the means are (approximately) normal.

Distribution of the difference between two independent sample means, $\bar{x}_1 - \bar{x}_2$

1. Mean, $\mu_{\bar{x}_1 - \bar{x}_2} = \mu_{\bar{x}_1} - \mu_{\bar{x}_2}$.
2. Variance, $\sigma^2_{\bar{x}_1 - \bar{x}_2} = \sigma^2_{\bar{x}_1} + \sigma^2_{\bar{x}_2}$.
3. Standard error, $\sigma_{\bar{x}_1 - \bar{x}_2} = \sqrt{\sigma^2_{\bar{x}_1} + \sigma^2_{\bar{x}_2}}$.
4. The distribution is (approximately) normal if both sampling distributions of the means are (approximately) normal.

The results for the sampling distributions of a sum and a difference are expressed in the context of the sample mean but may be generalised for any other statistic, such as the sample correlation coefficient or the sample proportion.

The distribution of the sample proportion, p

The population proportion, π, of individuals possessing a certain characteristic may be estimated by the sample proportion $p = r/n$, where the sample size is n of whom r individuals possess the characteristic. The distribution of the sample proportion is determined by computing the sample proportions ($p_1, p_2, \ldots, p_k$) for all possible samples of size n which can be drawn from the population. The sampling distribution of p has the following properties:

1. Mean, $\mu_p = \pi$.
2. Variance, $\sigma^2_p = \pi(1-\pi)/n$.

3. Standard error [SE(p)], $\sigma_p = \sqrt{\dfrac{\pi(1-\pi)}{n}}$.

4. The distribution is binomial. For reasonably large samples ($n \geq 30$, say), the binomial distribution may be approximated by the normal distribution.

The chi-square (χ^2) distribution

The χ^2 (the Greek letter, pronounced 'khi', squared) distribution is the sampling distribution of the statistic $X^2 = z_1^2 + z_2^2 + \ldots + z_\nu^2$ where $z_1, z_2, \ldots, z_\nu$ are independently distributed standard normal variables. The χ^2 distribution is a continuous distribution with the following properties:

1. The probability density function (which need not be memorised) is

$$p(\chi^2) = \chi_0^2 \exp(-\chi^2/2)(\chi^2)^{(\nu-2)/2} \qquad (0 \leq \chi^2)$$

where χ_0^2 is a constant depending on ν.

2. Characterised by ν (the Greek letter, nu), the *degrees of freedom*. The notation χ_ν^2 thus fully describes the distribution.

3. Positively skewed. As n increases, the curve approaches symmetry.

4. If x is normally distributed with variance σ^2 and estimated variance $s^2 = \sum(x_i - \bar{x})^2/(n-1)$ based on a sample of size n, then $(n-1)s^2/\sigma^2$ has a χ^2 distribution on $n-1$ degrees of freedom. The *sampling distribution of* s^2, when x is normally distributed, is thus $[\sigma^2/(n-1)]\chi_{(n-1)}^2$. The mean of the distribution is σ^2 and the variance is $2\sigma^4/(n-1)$.

5. The percentage point or critical value of χ^2, beyond which lies a specified percentage, $100\alpha\%$, of the total area enclosed by the probability density function, $p(\chi^2)$, and the horizontal axis, χ^2, is written here as $\chi_\nu^2(\alpha)$. The percentage points for different values of α and ν are tabulated (Table A2) (see also Fig. 5.1).

Student *t*-distribution

The *t*-distribution is the sampling distribution of the variable $t = z/\sqrt{(y/\nu)}$ where z is a standard normal variable, independent of the variable y which is distributed χ_ν^2. The *t*-distribution is a continuous distribution with the following properties:

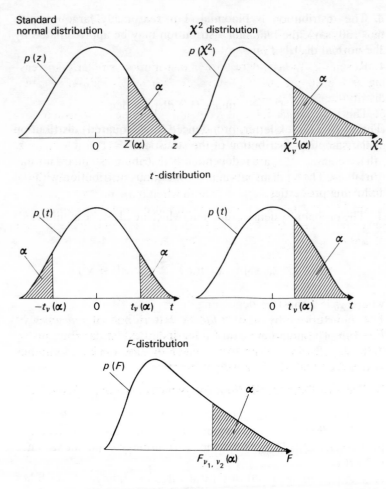

Fig. 5.1. Tabulated percentage points for some common distributions. The shaded tail areas are the corresponding tabulated probabilities.

1. The probability density function (which need not be memorised) is

$$p(t) = \frac{t_0}{\left(1 + \dfrac{t^2}{\nu}\right)^{(\nu+1)/2}} \qquad (-\infty < t < +\infty)$$

where t_0 is a constant depending on ν.

2. Characterised by v, the degrees of freedom. The notation t_v thus fully describes the distribution.

3. Symmetric about zero.

4. Resembles the standard normal distribution, similarity increasing as the sample size, n, increases. When n is infinite, the two distributions are identical.

5. The percentage point of t beyond which lies a specified percentage, $100\alpha\%$, of the total area enclosed by the probability density function, $p(t)$, and the horizontal axis, t, is written here as $t_v(\alpha)$. Since the t-distribution is symmetric about zero, $t_v(\alpha) = -t_v(1-\alpha)$. The percentage points for different values of α and v are tabulated (Table A3) both when only the upper tail area is considered ($100\alpha\%$ in one tail) and also when both upper and lower tail areas are considered ($100\alpha\%$ in each tail, giving a total of $200\alpha\%$ in both tails) (see also Fig. 5.1).

The F-distribution

The F-distribution is the sampling distribution of the variable $F = (u/v_1)/(v/v_2)$, where u and v are independent variables distributed as $\chi^2_{v_1}$ and $\chi^2_{v_2}$, respectively. The F-distribution is a continuous distribution with the following properties:

1. The probability density function (which need not be memorised) is

$$p(F) = F_0 \frac{F^{(v_1-2)/2}}{\left(1+\dfrac{v_1}{v_2} F\right)^{(v_1+v_2)/2}} \quad (F > 0)$$

where F_0 is a constant depending on v_1 and v_2.

2. Characterised by v_1 and v_1, the degrees of freedom. The notation F_{v_1,v_2} thus fully describes the distribution.

3. Positively skewed.

4. $F_{v_1,v_2} = t^2_{v_2}$.

5. The percentage point of F beyond which lies a specified percentage, $100\alpha\%$, of the total area enclosed by the probability density function, $p(F)$, and the horizontal axis, F, is written here as $F_{v_1,v_2}(\alpha)$. The percentage points for different values of v_1, v_2 and α are tabulated (Table A4) (see also Fig. 5.1).

Examples

Distribution of the sample mean

Assume that the MCV (mean corpuscular volume) in a community of adults is normally distributed with mean $\mu = 86$ μm^3 and standard deviation $\sigma = 4$ μm^3. If random samples each of 25 adults are obtained, the mean ($\mu_{\bar{x}}$) and its standard error ($\sigma_{\bar{x}}$) of the resulting normal sampling distribution of means of MCV are respectively:

$$\text{and } \begin{aligned} \mu_{\bar{x}} &= \mu = 86 \ \mu m^3 \\ \sigma_{\bar{x}} &= \sigma/\sqrt{n} = 4/\sqrt{25} = 0.8 \ \mu m^3. \end{aligned}$$

Distribution of the difference between two independent sample means

Assume that the distribution of daily Calorie intake (kcal/day) in boys aged 1–2 years has mean $\mu_1 = 1287$ and standard deviation $\sigma_1 = 198$ and that the distribution in boys aged 2–3 years has mean $\mu_2 = 1403$ and standard deviation $\sigma_2 = 205$. If independent random samples of 27 boys aged 1–2 years and 25 boys aged 2–3 years are obtained, the mean ($\mu_{\bar{x}_1-\bar{x}_2}$) and its standard error ($\sigma_{\bar{x}_1-\bar{x}_2}$) of the sampling distribution of the difference between the mean Calorie intake in boys in the two age groups are respectively:

$$\mu_{\bar{x}_1-\bar{x}_2} = \mu_{\bar{x}_1} - \mu_{\bar{x}_2} = \mu_1 - \mu_2 = 1287 - 1403 = -116 \text{ kcal/day}$$

and

$$\sigma_{\bar{x}_1-\bar{x}_2} = \sqrt{\sigma_{\bar{x}_1}^2 + \sigma_{\bar{x}_2}^2} = \sqrt{\frac{\sigma_1^2}{27} + \frac{\sigma_2^2}{25}} = \sqrt{\frac{198^2}{27} + \frac{205^2}{25}}$$
$$= \sqrt{3133} = 56 \text{ kcal/day}.$$

Distribution of the sample proportion

In a population of 5-year-old schoolchildren, 20% possess the sickle cell trait. It is of interest to determine the standard error of the proportion (p) of sicklers in repeated samples of 150 from this population of schoolchildren.

$\pi = 0.2$, the true proportion of sicklers in the population

$n = 150$

$\text{Var}(p) = \pi(1-\pi)/n = (0.2)(1-0.2)/150 = 0.001$

$\text{SE}(p) = \sqrt{0.001} = 0.033.$

Chapter 6
Estimation

Introduction

A sample statistic (e.g. $\bar{x}$) may estimate a true but unknown population parameter (e.g. μ), but its worth as an estimator is questionable without some statement of its precision. Thus it is necessary to quote either:

1. The **standard error** of the estimate in addition to the sample statistic which estimates the population parameter. The number of observations in the sample, n, should also be indicated to enhance judgement on reliability.

If the sample *mean* is used to estimate the population mean, the standard deviation of the observations may be quoted instead of the standard error of the mean, since the two are directly related by $\sqrt{n}$ (see Chapter 5). It should be noted that the standard error of the mean and the standard deviation have distinct and separate roles. The standard deviation is a measure of the spread of the observations and should be reported with the estimated mean when the aim is to describe the distribution of the data. The standard error of the mean relates to the precision of the estimated mean and should be reported when attention is centred on the mean; e.g. when one mean is compared with another.

2. A **confidence interval** for the population parameter. This is the interval (generally symmetric about the sample statistic which estimates the population parameter) containing the unknown true value of the parameter with a known probability. The probabilities usually chosen are 0.99, 0.95 and 0.90 leading to 99%, 95% and 90% confidence intervals, respectively.

Confidence intervals are discussed for the population mean (μ), standard deviation (σ) and proportion (π). The 95% confidence intervals for these parameters are summarised in Table 6.1. It is *assumed* in calculating confidence intervals for μ and σ that the variable x is *normally* distributed with mean μ and variance σ^2. A random sample of n observations, $x_1, x_2, \ldots, x_n$, is selected from the population.

47

Table 6.1 95% confidence intervals for various parameters

Parameter	Conditions	95% confidence interval
Mean, μ	x dist. $N(\mu, \sigma^2)$ (i) σ known	$\left(\bar{x}-1.96\dfrac{\sigma}{\sqrt{n}},\ \bar{x}+1.96\dfrac{\sigma}{\sqrt{n}}\right)$
	(ii) σ unknown, n large	$\left(\bar{x}-1.96\dfrac{s}{\sqrt{n}},\ \bar{x}+1.96\dfrac{s}{\sqrt{n}}\right)$
	(iii) σ unknown, n small	$\left(\bar{x}-t_{n-1}(0.025)\dfrac{s}{\sqrt{n}},\right.$ $\left.\bar{x}+t_{n-1}(0.025)\dfrac{s}{\sqrt{n}}\right)$
Proportion, π	n large (i) without continuity correction	$\left(p-1.96\sqrt{\dfrac{pq}{n}},\ p+1.96\sqrt{\dfrac{pq}{n}}\right)$
	(ii) with continuity correction	$\left(p-\dfrac{1}{2n}-1.96\sqrt{\dfrac{pq}{n}},\right.$ $\left.p+\dfrac{1}{2n}+1.96\sqrt{\dfrac{pq}{n}}\right)$
Standard deviation, σ	x dist. $N(\mu, \sigma^2)$	$\left(\dfrac{s\sqrt{n-1}}{\chi_{n-1}(0.025)},\ \dfrac{s\sqrt{n-1}}{\chi_{n-1}(0.975)}\right)$

$\bar{x} = \sum x_i/n,\ s = \sqrt{\sum (x_i-\bar{x})^2/(n-1)}, p = r/n,\ q = 1-p.$

95% confidence interval for the population mean, μ

The sample mean, $\bar{x} = \sum x_i/n$, is an unbiased estimator of μ. If x is distributed $N(\mu, \sigma^2)$ then $\bar{x}$ is distributed $N(\mu, \sigma^2/n)$ (see Chapter 5). The form of the confidence interval for μ depends on whether σ^2 is known or unknown.

Population variance, σ^2, known

A 95% confidence interval for μ is the interval from $\bar{x}-1.96\sigma/\sqrt{n}$ to

$\bar{x}+1.96\sigma/\sqrt{n}$, written $(\bar{x}-1.96\sigma/\sqrt{n}, \bar{x}+1.96\sigma/\sqrt{n})$. That is,

$$\Pr\left(\bar{x}-1.96\frac{\sigma}{\sqrt{n}} < \mu < \bar{x}+1.96\frac{\sigma}{\sqrt{n}}\right) = 0.95.$$

This is a central confidence interval, symmetric about $\bar{x}$, such that in the long run there is a 2.5% chance that μ is greater than the *upper confidence limit* of $\bar{x}+1.96\sigma/\sqrt{n}$ and a 2.5% chance that μ is less than the *lower confidence limit* of $\bar{x}-1.96\sigma/\sqrt{n}$. The percentage confidence, in this instance of 95%, is called the *confidence level* or the *confidence coefficient*. The number 1.96, corresponding to a 95% confidence level, is called the *critical value* and is obtained from tables of the standard normal distribution (Table A1). The critical value changes as the confidence level alters. The 99%, 95% and 90% confidence levels are most commonly employed in practice and have corresponding critical values of 2.58, 1.96 (often approximated by 2.00) and 1.645, respectively. A critical value of 1.00 corresponds to a confidence level of 68%.

Justification

It is stated (Chapter 4) that if a random variable x is distributed $N(\mu, \sigma^2)$, then

$$\Pr(\mu-1.96\sigma < x < \mu+1.96\sigma) = 0.95.$$

Thus, similarly, if $\bar{x}$ is distributed $N(\mu, \sigma^2/n)$, then

$$\Pr\left(\mu-1.96\frac{\sigma}{\sqrt{n}} < \bar{x} < \mu+1.96\frac{\sigma}{\sqrt{n}}\right) = 0.95. \qquad (6.1)$$

Equation (6.1) justifies a probability interval for $\bar{x}$ (known) dependent on knowledge of μ (unknown). Since the requirement is for an interval for μ (unknown) calculated from $\bar{x}$ (known), the inequalities within the probabilistic identity of equation (6.1) may be rearranged to produce the required interval.

The *relation* between the confidence level, the critical value and the standard normal distribution may be explained if it is remembered that if $\bar{x}$ is distributed $N(\mu, \sigma^2/n)$, then the standard normal deviate of $\bar{x}$, $z = (\bar{x}-\mu)/(\sigma/\sqrt{n})$, is distributed $N(0, 1)$.

Hence

$$\Pr\left(\bar{x} - 1.96\,\frac{\sigma}{\sqrt{n}} < \mu < \bar{x} + 1.96\,\frac{\sigma}{\sqrt{n}}\right)$$

$$= \Pr\left(\mu < \bar{x} + 1.96\,\frac{\sigma}{\sqrt{n}}\right) - \Pr\left(\mu < \bar{x} - 1.96\,\frac{\sigma}{\sqrt{n}}\right)$$

$$= \Pr\left(\frac{\bar{x} - \mu}{\sigma/\sqrt{n}} < 1.96\right) - \Pr\left(\frac{\bar{x} - \mu}{\sigma/\sqrt{n}} > 1.96\right)$$

$$= 0.975 - 0.025$$

$$= 0.95.$$

This probability is the shaded area in Fig. 6.1.

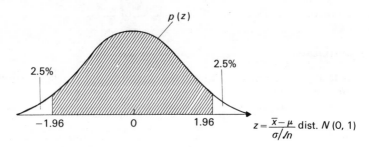

Fig. 6.1 The standard normal distribution.

Population variance, σ^2, unknown

The confidence interval for the mean μ is based on the standard normal deviate, $z = (\bar{x} - \mu)/(\sigma/\sqrt{n})$, in which σ is known. If σ is unknown, it is replaced by the sample estimator

$$s = \sqrt{\sum(x_i - \bar{x})^2/(n-1)}.$$

1. *n large,* $(n \geqslant 30, \; say)$

The sampling distribution of the statistic $(\bar{x} - \mu)/(s/\sqrt{n})$ is approximately standard normal when n is large. The confidence interval for μ when σ is unknown and n is large then differs from that in which σ is known, only in σ, which is replaced by s. Thus the 95% confidence interval for μ when σ is unknown is

$$\left(\bar{x}-1.96\frac{s}{\sqrt{n}}, \ \bar{x}+1.96\frac{s}{\sqrt{n}}\right).$$

2. *n small, (n < 30, say)*
The sampling distribution of the statistic $(\bar{x}-\mu)/(s/\sqrt{n})$ is not normal when n is small, but it is a *t*-distribution on $n-1$ degrees of freedom. The confidence interval for μ in this instance differs from that in which σ is known, not only in σ but also in its critical value. The critical value is now the appropriate percentage point of the *t*-distribution and not of the standard normal distribution. In general terms, the critical value for a $100(1-2\alpha)\%$ confidence interval for μ symmetric about the sample mean when σ is unknown is $t_{n-1}(\alpha)$. Thus, in particular, for a 95% confidence interval for μ when σ is unknown, the critical value is $t_{n-1}(0.025)$ and the confidence interval is

$$\left(\bar{x}-t_{n-1}(0.025)\frac{s}{\sqrt{n}}, \ \bar{x}+t_{n-1}(0.025)\frac{s}{\sqrt{n}}\right).$$

Note: The number 30 is used here to distinguish large n from small n. It should be stressed that the choice of this number is arbitrary and should be dependent on the nature of the data. The quantity 30 provides only a guideline. Furthermore, the tables of the *t*-distribution provide percentage points for large as well as small n. Thus a simple approach to determining a confidence interval for μ is always to obtain the critical value from tables of the *t*-distribution corresponding to the true sampling distribution of the statistic $(\bar{x}-\mu)/(s/\sqrt{n})$.

95% confidence interval for a population proportion, π

The population proportion, π, of individuals possessing a certain characteristic may be estimated by the sample proportion $p = r/n$, where the sample size is n of whom r individuals possess the characteristic. The sampling distribution of p is binomial which may be approximated by the normal distribution for large enough $n(n \geqslant 30)$. The standard deviation of the sampling distribution of p is $\sqrt{\pi(1-\pi)/n}$ which may be approximated by $\sqrt{p(1-p)/n}$ since

π is unknown. Thus

$$z = (p-\pi)/\sqrt{p(1-p)/n}$$

is approximately normally distributed with zero mean and unit variance, and so the critical value is obtained from standard normal tables (Table A1). The critical value corresponding to a 95% confidence level is 1.96. The 95% confidence interval for π symmetric about p is thus

$$\left(p-1.96\sqrt{\frac{pq}{n}},\ p+1.96\sqrt{\frac{pq}{n}}\right)$$

where $q = 1-p$. With the continuity correction, the 95% confidence interval for π is

$$\left(p-\frac{1}{2n}-1.96\sqrt{\frac{pq}{n}},\ p+\frac{1}{2n}+1.96\sqrt{\frac{pq}{n}}\right).$$

95% confidence interval for a population standard deviation, σ

The sample statistic $s^2 = \sum(x_i-\bar{x})^2/(n-1)$ is an unbiased estimator of the population variance, σ^2. If x is distributed $N(\mu,\ \sigma^2)$, the statistic $(n-1)s^2/\sigma^2$ has a χ^2 distribution on $n-1$ degrees of freedom (see Chapter 5). Hence, using the tables of the χ^2 distribution (Table A2), it is possible to find two percentage points, $\chi^2_{n-1}(0.025)$ and $\chi^2_{n-1}(0.975)$, such that

$$\Pr\left[\chi^2_{n-1}(0.975) < \frac{(n-1)s^2}{\sigma^2} < \chi^2_{n-1}(0.025)\right] = 0.95,$$

or equivalently,

$$\Pr\left[\frac{s\sqrt{n-1}}{\chi_{n-1}(0.025)} < \sigma < \frac{s\sqrt{n-1}}{\chi_{n-1}(0.975)}\right] = 0.95.$$

Thus the 95% confidence interval for σ is

$$\left(\frac{s\sqrt{n-1}}{\chi_{n-1}(0.025)},\ \frac{s\sqrt{n-1}}{\chi_{n-1}(0.975)}\right).$$

It should be noted that since the χ^2 distribution is asymmetric,

$$\chi_{n-1}(0.025) \neq \chi_{n-1}(0.975).$$

Also, these intervals tend to be relatively large.

Normal range

In medicine, it is often of interest to determine not only the *confidence interval* for a population parameter (the interval which contains the true value of the parameter with a specified probability) but also the *normal range* of the observations (the interval within which the value of an observation on an individual should lie in order that the individual be considered 'normal'). Generally the normal range is that interval which contains the central 95% of the observations in the population. Then it is unlikely (the chance of such an eventuality is at most 5%) that the value of an observation on an individual who is 'normal' with respect to the variable of interest lies outside the normal range.

If the variable of interest is approximately normally distributed with true mean μ and variance σ^2, then (see Chapter 4) approximately 95% of the observations are contained in the interval $\mu \pm 2\sigma$. This interval, $(\mu - 2\sigma, \mu + 2\sigma)$, is the normal range. In practice, it is rarely feasible to examine the whole population and a very large sample suffices (unfortunately, all too often, a fallacious normal range is determined, being derived from a 'very large' sample of only 30 or 40 instead of at least hundreds of observations).

Note: There is a distinction between the use of 'normal' in statistical terminology referring to the Gaussian distribution and in the non-statistician's concept of the term.

Examples

95% confidence interval for the population mean, μ

A random sample of 11 subjects is selected from a population. The following figures are the values of the variable, x, the clotting time (min) of plasma, for these 11 individuals.

7.9, 10.9, 11.3, 11.9, 15.0, 12.7, 12.3, 8.6, 9.4, 11.3, 11.5.

$n = 11$
$\bar{x} = 122.8/11 = 11.16$
$s^2 = \sum(x_i - \bar{x})^2/(11-1) = 39.47/10 = 3.95$
$s = 1.99.$

Population variance, σ^2, known

Suppose (this is very unlikely) that it is known in advance that the standard deviation of the distribution of the clotting time of plasma, σ, is 1.87 min. The 95% confidence interval for μ, the true mean clotting time of plasma, is the interval

$$(\bar{x}-1.96\sigma/\sqrt{n}, \bar{x}+1.96\sigma/\sqrt{n}) = [11.16-(1.96)(1.87)/\sqrt{11},$$
$$11.16+(1.96)(1.87)/\sqrt{11}]$$
$$= (11.16-1.11, 11.16+1.11)$$
$$= (10.05, 12.27) \text{ min.}$$

Thus the probability is 0.95 that the interval 10.05–12.27 min contains the true mean clotting time of plasma.

Population variance, σ^2, unknown

The 95% confidence interval for μ is

$$[\bar{x}-t_{n-1}(0.025)s/\sqrt{n}, \bar{x}+t_{n-1}(0.025)s/\sqrt{n}]$$
$$= [11.16-(2.23)(1.99)/\sqrt{11}, 11.16+(2.23)(1.99)/\sqrt{11}]$$
$$= (11.16-1.34, 11.16+1.34)$$
$$= (9.82, 12.50) \text{ min.}$$

95% confidence interval for a population proportion, π

A large number of mites are placed on a cotton rat with microfilarial infection. After a certain time 50 mites (assumed to be effectively a random sample from the whole population) are dissected and 10 found to be infected. The observed proportion of infected mites, $p = 10/50 = 0.2$, is thus an estimate of π, the true proportion of infected mites in the population. The 95% confidence interval for π is

$$\left[p-1.96\sqrt{\frac{p(1-p)}{n}}, p+1.96\sqrt{\frac{p(1-p)}{n}}\right]$$
$$= \left[0.2-1.96\sqrt{\frac{(0.2)(0.8)}{50}}, 0.2+1.96\sqrt{\frac{(0.2)(0.8)}{50}}\right]$$
$$= (0.2-0.11, 0.2+0.11)$$
$$= (0.09, 0.31).$$

More correctly, with the continuity correction, the 95% confidence interval for π is

$$\left[p - \frac{1}{100} - 1.96\sqrt{\frac{p(1-p)}{n}}, \; p + \frac{1}{100} + 1.96\sqrt{\frac{p(1-p)}{n}} \right]$$

$$= (0.09 - 0.01, \; 0.31 + 0.01)$$
$$= (0.08, \; 0.32).$$

95% confidence interval for a population standard deviation, σ

Using the sample data of the clotting time of plasma (min) in 11 subjects

$$s^2 = 3.95 \qquad \chi^2_{10}(0.025) = 20.48, \qquad \chi_{10}(0.025) = 4.53$$
$$s = 1.99 \qquad \chi^2_{10}(0.975) = 3.25, \qquad \chi_{10}(0.975) = 1.80$$
$$n = 11.$$

The 95% confidence interval for σ, the standard deviation of the distribution of the clotting time of plasma, is the interval

$$\left[\frac{s\sqrt{n-1}}{\chi_{n-1}(0.025)}, \; \frac{s\sqrt{n-1}}{\chi_{n-1}(0.975)} \right] = \left[\frac{(1.99)\sqrt{10}}{4.53}, \; \frac{(1.99)\sqrt{10}}{1.80} \right]$$

$$= \left(\frac{6.29}{4.53}, \frac{6.29}{1.80} \right)$$

$$= (1.39, \; 3.49) \text{ min.}$$

Note: This confidence interval is asymmetric about s and is large.

Chapter 7
Tests of Hypotheses

Introduction

Chapter 6 dealt with the *estimation* of population parameters by sample statistics. These sample statistics may be further utilised to answer *questions* about the population parameters. In the framework of statistical inference, the question is reduced to an hypothesis and the answer to it expressed as the result of a test of the hypothesis. The investigator forms an opinion on the basis of this test and generally is prompted into making a decision resulting in some form of action.

Approach

Statement

In simplest terms, the requirement is for an answer to a question concerning the value of a population parameter (e.g. μ). The procedure is to formulate the question in such a way that there are only two answers to it: yes or no (e.g. $\mu = 0$?). Then the interrogative content is extracted from the question so that it is replaced by a statement (null hypothesis) specifying the value of the parameter (e.g. $\mu = 0$); this statement may be true or false.

Test

A random sample of observations is taken and the following question asked: 'To what extent do the observations in the sample throw light on the plausibility of the statement?' If the results observed in the sample differ markedly (evaluated probabilistically) from those expected if the statement were true (as judged through the concepts of sampling theory by consideration of a test statistic and its critical region), then the observed differences are said to be *significant* and the statement is rejected as a reasonable description of the situation. The whole procedure is called a test of significance or a test of hypothesis.

Error

It is possible to come to the wrong conclusion regarding the truth of the statement. The two possible errors are: (i) to reject the statement when it is true (Type I error); and (ii) not to reject the statement when it is false (Type II error) (see Table 7.1). Ideally, a 'good' test is one in which both of these errors are as small as possible. In reality, simultaneous minimisation of both of these errors is difficult, if not impossible. Generally, the Type I error is considered to be of prime importance, and the probability associated with it (the significance level) is fixed, and that test chosen which then minimises the probability associated with the Type II

Table 7.1 Errors associated with a statistical statement, H_0

	Reject H_0	Do not reject H_0
H_0 true	Type I error	No error
H_0 false	No error	Type II error

error. Equally, if consideration is given to one minus the probability associated with the Type II error (the *power* of the test, for a specified alternative value of the parameter under test, expressing the probability of rejecting the null hypothesis when it is false and the alternative value prevails), then a 'good' test is one which, for a fixed significance level, maximises the power of the test. Sometimes the power function curve (i.e. the power plotted against various alternative values of the parameter under test) is examined to aid comparison of several procedures for performing tests of significance. The choice of test to satisfy the above-mentioned criteria is not discussed further. The tests described are those which have been shown theoretically to be 'good'.

Terminology

Statistical hypothesis

This is a statement about the parameter(s) or distributional form of the population(s) being sampled.

Null hypothesis, H_0

In general, this term relates to the particular hypothesis under test. In many instances it is formulated for the sole purpose of being rejected or nullified. It is often an hypothesis of 'no difference'.

Alternative hypothesis, H_1

This is a statistical hypothesis that disagrees with the null hypothesis.

Type I error

If, as the result of a statistical test, a statistical hypothesis is rejected when it ought not to be rejected (i.e. when it is true), then an error of the first kind (Type I error) is committed.

Type II error

If, as the result of a statistical test, a statistical hypothesis is not rejected when it is false (i.e. when it should have been rejected), then an error of the second kind (Type II error) is committed.

Test statistic

This is a mathematical function (expression) of sample values which provides a basis for testing a statistical hypothesis. It is chosen theoretically to satisfy certain 'error' criteria and generally has a known sampling distribution with tabulated percentage points (e.g. standard normal, χ^2, t, F).

Significance level (α)

This is the probability associated with a Type I error; i.e. the probability of rejecting H_0 when it is true. The significance level is often expressed as a percentage, i.e. the probability, α, is multiplied by 100. If the significance level is chosen at the outset of the test, it expresses the risk the investigator is prepared to accept of committing a Type I error. Often the 5%, 1% and 0.1% (i.e. $\alpha = 0.05, 0.01, 0.001$, respectively) levels are chosen as important, but the selection is fairly arbitrary and should depend on the particular problem and its interpretation.

Critical (rejection) region

This is a set of values of the test statistic leading to rejection of the null hypothesis. If the value of the test statistic computed from the sample lies within the range of values specified as the critical region, then the null hypothesis is rejected. The location of the critical region is dependent on the sampling distribution of the test statistic and the significance level specification.

Critical value

This is the value of the test statistic corresponding to a given significance level as determined from the sampling distribution of the test statistic. If the value of the test statistic computed from the sample data is *equal* to the critical value, H_0 is rejected and the probability of an error (Type I error) occurring as a result of this action is *equal* to the significance level. The critical value is the boundary value of the critical region such that if the value of the test statistic is *more extreme* than the critical value, then H_0 is rejected and the probability of an error occurring as a result of this action is *less* than the significance level.

Critical level (*P* value)

The critical level, commonly called the *P* value, provides a more precise statement of the findings about the propriety of H_0 than the significance level. It is the maximum probability of rejecting H_0 when H_0 is true, in the observed situation. Determining the critical level is an alternative to declaring a significance level at the outset of the test, and deciding to reject H_0 if the observed value of the test statistic falls in the critical region determined by the significance level.

Significant value of the test statistic

This is a value of the test statistic falling into the critical region, leading to rejection of H_0. Generally, when a sample produces a value of the test statistic in the critical region, the results are said to be statistically significant. Note the distinction between the layman's interpretation of significant meaning important (noticeable, considerable, substantial, meaningful, etc.) and the statistical interpretation with its probabilistic and error connotations.

Test of hypothesis

This is a procedure whereby the truth of a null hypothesis is investigated by examining the value of the test statistic computed from a sample. The decision is taken to reject H_0 at a given level of significance if this computed value falls in the critical region determined by the significance level specification.

Figure 7.1 illustrates the relationship between some of the terms described and the sampling distribution of the test statistic when H_0 is true. Only one tail of the sampling distribution is considered.

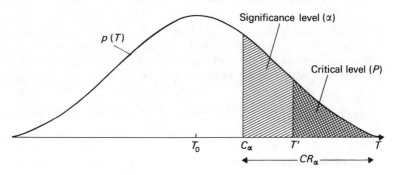

Fig. 7.1 Sampling distribution of the test statistic, T, when H_0 is true. T_0, value of T under H_0. C_α, critical value corresponding to a significance level of α; CR_α, critical region corresponding to a significance level of α; T', computed value of T, lying in CR_α and leading to rejection of $H_0(P < \alpha)$; $p(T)$, probability density function of T.

Procedure

The procedure is considered in the simplest case when a single parameter is under test but it is appropriate with only minor modifications when more complex hypotheses are investigated.

1. Specify the **null hypothesis,** H_0
Generally when the hypothesis relates to:
　　a. A single parameter from one population (e.g. μ), H_0 specifies a value for the parameter (e.g. H_0: $\mu = 0$);
　　b. The same parameter in $k > 1$ populations (e.g. μ_1, μ_2, . . . , μ_k), H_0 is stated in terms of 'no difference' in the values

of the parameter in the populations (e.g. $k = 2$, H_0: $\mu_1 = \mu_2$ or $\mu_1 - \mu_2 = 0$).

2. Specify the **alternative hypothesis,** H_1, *before* the data are gathered, on the basis of the results expected theoretically (in biological terms) or from previous experience. This specification determines whether the test is *one-tailed* or *two-tailed*. In particular, suppose P is a parameter (e.g. $P = \mu$ or $P = \mu_1 - \mu_2$) and P_0 any value (e.g. $P_0 = 0$). Then the alternative hypothesis may be one of the following:

    a. H_1^i: $P \neq P_0$

i.e. if H_0 is false, a difference exists between P and P_0, but its direction is uncertain; either $P > P_0$ or $P < P_0$. This leads to a two-tailed test.

    b. H_1^{ii}: $P > P_0$

i.e. if H_0 is false, a difference exists between P and P_0 and its direction is known. This leads to a one-tailed test.

    c. H_1^{iii}: $P < P_0$

i.e. if H_0 is false, a difference exists between P and P_0 and its direction is known. This leads to a one-tailed test.

In general, particularly at the start of a statistical investigation, there is considerable doubt as to the direction of a difference. Hence a two-tailed test is most commonly appropriate, and is thus described in this work more fully than its counterpart.

The distinction between one- and two-tailed tests is relevant to the choice of critical region, as described in step 7.

3. Collect a random sample of data from the population(s).

4. Plot the sample data to give an indication of the distribution of the data and the conclusions that may be drawn from the data. The form of the diagram depends on the nature of the data and the null hypothesis specification.

5. Determine the appropriate **test statistic,** T, and its sampling distribution under H_0 (when H_0 is true), generally by considering:

    a. The sample statistic which estimates the parameter under test.

    b. The sampling distribution of this statistic and, if applicable, the sampling distribution of the difference in two such statistics.

    c. A transformation, if necessary, of this statistic or the difference in two statistics, as appropriate, to a new statistic which embodies all parameters under test, and whose sampling distribution has tabulated percentage points (e.g. standard normal, χ^2, t, F).

d. The parameter specification of H_0 which is incorporated into the new statistic to produce the test statistic.

6. Compute the value, T_C, of the test statistic using the sample data.

7. Determine the **critical region** of values of the test statistic associated with a specified significance level.

Location of the critical region

The location (determined by the appropriate percentage point, C_α, of the sampling distribution of T) but not the size of the critical region is dependent on whether the test is one- or two-tailed (determined by the specification of H_1). In a one-tailed test, the critical region is entirely at one end (or tail) of the sampling distribution of the test statistic. In a two-tailed test, the critical region is located at both ends of the sampling distribution.

Determination of appropriate percentage points to define the critical region

In general terms:

a. *If the sampling distribution of T is $N(0, 1)$ or t_ν*
The critical region for a *two-tailed* test at the $200\alpha\%$ level of significance is the set of values of the test statistic so large or so small that when H_0 is true, the probability associated with their occurrence is at most 2α. Thus if C_α is the critical value obtained from tables corresponding to the sampling distribution of the test statistic $[C_\alpha = Z(\alpha)$ *or* $C_\alpha = t_\nu(\alpha)]$ such that $100\alpha\%$ of the total probability is contained in each tail of the symmetric distribution, then the critical region is the set of values of T greater than C_α and less than $-C_\alpha$. Alternatively expressed, the critical region is the set of *absolute* values of T greater than C_α (the *absolute* value of T, written $|T|$, is the value of T without regard to sign).

b. *If the sampling distribution of T is χ^2_ν or F_{ν_1, ν_2}*
Generally (one exception discussed in Chapter 8 is the test for equality of variances) only the upper tail of the sampling distribution of T is of issue. The critical region for a test at the

$100\alpha\%$ level of significance is then the set of values of T greater C_α, where C_α is the critical value obtained from tables corresponding to the sampling distribution of the test statistic $[C_\alpha = \chi^2_v(\alpha)$ or $C_\alpha = F_{v_1, v_2}(\alpha)]$ such that $100\alpha\%$ of the total probability is contained in the upper tail of the distribution.

Rejection procedure

Reject H_0 at the specified level of significance if the computed value, T_C, of the test statistic falls in the critical region, and *do not reject* H_0 otherwise.

Rejection terminology

Although rejection of H_0 is a feasible consequence of a 'significant' result in that there is sufficient evidence provided against H_0, a 'non-significant' result should *not* precipitate the acceptance of H_0. A non-significant result does not provide positive evidence in favour of H_0 but rather it indicates a *lack* of strong evidence against H_0. Thus, in this situation, it is more appropriate *not to reject* H_0 than to accept it.

Hypothesis tests of a population mean, μ

The variable x is normally distributed in the population with mean μ and variance σ^2. Two situations are considered: (i) σ^2 known (from previous experience); and (ii) σ^2 unknown.

σ^2 known

The test of a population mean (σ^2 known) is described but the procedure is applicable, with a change only in notation, to a test of any parameter which is estimated by a statistic whose sampling distribution is normal. The procedure is:

1. Specify H_0: $\mu = \mu_0$, where μ_0 is a particular value.
2. Specify H_1: $\mu \neq \mu_0$, say.
3. Select a random sample of observations, $x_1, x_2, \ldots, x_n$.
4. Plot these observations along a single scale of values. Consider the position of μ_0 in relation to these values. The distribution of these observations should be approximately normal in order that

the remaining steps be valid. An illustration is given in Fig. 7.2.

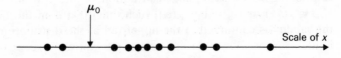

Fig. 7.2 Plot of (hypothetical) sample observations for H_0: $\mu = \mu_0$.

5. Consider the test statistic

$$T_1 = (\bar{x} - \mu_0)/(\sigma/\sqrt{n})$$

where $\bar{x} = \sum x_i/n$. The sampling distribution of T_1 is approximately standard normal. T_1 is chosen because:

    a. The sample statistic which estimates the parameter under test, μ, is the sample mean, $\bar{x}$.

    b. The sampling distribution of $\bar{x}$ is $N(\mu, \sigma^2/n)$.

    c. The sampling distribution of $(\bar{x} - \mu)/(\sigma/\sqrt{n})$ is $N(0, 1)$ which has tabulated percentage points.

    d. The parameter specification of H_0 is $\mu = \mu_0$.

6. Compute the value, T_{1C}, of the test statistic from the sample data.

7. Determine the critical region from tables of the standard normal distribution (Table A1). Since the specification of H_1 has no direction, the critical region consists of both tails of the distribution. Thus for a two-tailed test at the $200\alpha\%$ level of significance, reject H_0 if $|T_{1C}| > Z(\alpha)$ [i.e. if $T_{1C} > Z(\alpha)$ or $T_{1C} < -Z(\alpha)$], $P < 2\alpha$. Do not reject H_0 otherwise, $P > 2\alpha$. In particular, if $2\alpha = 0.05$, 0.01 or 0.001, then $Z(\alpha) = 1.96$, 2.58 or 3.29, respectively.

σ^2 unknown

The more common situation is that in which the population variance, σ^2, is unknown and has to be estimated from the sample. Steps **1–4** are as previously described when σ^2 is known.

5. Consider the test statistic.

$$T_2 = (\bar{x} - \mu_0)/(s/\sqrt{n})$$

where $s = \sqrt{\sum(x_i - \bar{x})^2/(n-1)}$, the sample estimator of σ. This test statistic is a logical modification of T_1. Determination of the sampling distribution of T_2 depends on the size of the sample.

a. *n large ($\geq$ 30, say)*

T_2 has an approximately standard normal distribution. Thus the procedure (i.e. the remaining steps **6** and **7**) for testing H_0 is identical to that described when σ is known, except σ is replaced by s.

b. *n small ($n <$ 30, say)*

T_2 has a *t*-distribution on $n-1$ degrees of freedom. *Note:* As in Chapter 6 (confidence interval for μ; σ^2 unknown), the choice of n which distinguishes large from small n is arbitrary, and it is often simpler always to relate T_2 to the *t*-distribution, its true sampling distribution.

6. Compute the value, T_{2C}, of the test statistic from the sample data.

7. Determine the critical region from tables of the *t*-distribution (Table A3). For a two-tailed test at the $200\alpha\%$ level of significance, reject H_0 if $|T_{2C}| > t_{n-1}(\alpha)$ [i.e. if $T_{2C} > t_{n-1}(\alpha)$ or $T_{2C} < -t_{n-1}(\alpha)$], $P < 2\alpha$. Do not reject H_0 otherwise, $P > 2\alpha$.

The procedure for testing H_0: $\mu = \mu_0$ is summarised in the flowchart of Fig. 7.3.

Hypothesis test of a population proportion, π

Sometimes it is of interest to determine whether the proportion of individuals in the population, π, possessing some characteristic is equal to a particular value. Commonly this value is 1/2 in which case the proportions of individuals with and without the characteristic are equal. The procedure is to:

1. Specify H_0: $\pi = \pi_0$, where π_0 is a particular value.

2. Specify H_1: $\pi \neq \pi_0$, say.

3. Select a random sample of n individuals and determine the number, r, of them with the characteristic.

4. In this instance there is no way of illustrating the observations to aid interpretation. This step is thus waived.

5. Consider the test statistic

$$T_3 = (p - \pi_0)/\sqrt{\pi_0(1-\pi_0)/n}$$

where $p = r/n$. This test statistic has a standard normal distribution and is chosen because:

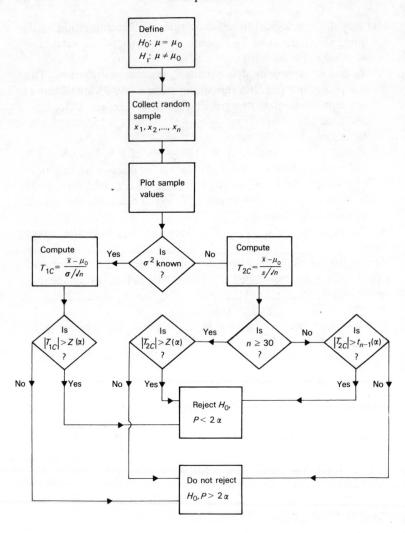

Fig. 7.3 Flow chart of the procedure for testing H_0: $\mu = \mu_0$ against H_1: $\mu \neq \mu_0$ when x dist. $N(\mu, \sigma^2)$, $\bar{x} = \sum x_i/n$, $s^2 = \sum (x_i - \bar{x})^2/(n-1)$.

a. The sample statistic which estimates the parameter under test is $p = r/n$, the sample proportion.

b. The sampling distribution of p is binomial which may be approximated by $N\{\pi, [\pi(1-\pi)/n]\}$ if n is large.

c. The sampling distribution of $(p-\pi)/\sqrt{\pi(1-\pi)/n}$ is standard normal which has tabulated percentage points.

d. The parameter specification of H_0 is $\pi = \pi_0$.

In practice, a continuity correction is applied to the test statistic to allow for the approximation of the discrete binomial distribution by the continuous normal distribution. The continuity correction is the subtraction of $1/(2n)$ from the absolute value (the value without regard to sign) of the numerator of the test statistic, i.e. take

$$T_3 = [|p-\pi_0|-1/(2n)]/\sqrt{\pi_0(1-\pi_0)/n}.$$

6. Compute the value, T_{3C}, of the test statistic from the sample data.

7. Determine the critical region from tables of the standard normal distribution (Table A1). For a two-tailed test at the $200\alpha\%$ level of significance, reject H_0 if $|T_{3C}| > Z(\alpha)$, $P < 2\alpha$. Do not reject H_0 otherwise, $P > 2\alpha$.

Examples

Hypothesis test of a population mean, μ

Let μ be the true mean clotting time (min) of plasma in the population. Let σ be the true standard deviation of the distribution of the clotting time of plasma.

1. H_0: $\mu = 10.0$.

2. H_1: $\mu \neq 10.0$, say.

3. A random sample of 11 individuals is selected. The clotting times of plasma of these individuals are 7.9, 10.9, 11.3, 11.9, 15.0, 12.7, 12.3, 8.6, 9.4, 11.3 and 11.5 min. (These are the same data as discussed in the Examples section of Chapter 6.)

4. The observations are plotted along a single scale of values as shown in Fig. E7.1. The data appear to be approximately normally distributed.

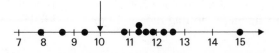

Fig. E7.1 Distribution of clotting times of plasma (min).

σ^2 known (very unlikely)

5. Consider

$$T_1 = (\bar{x} - \mu_0)/(\sigma/\sqrt{n})$$

where

$n = 11$
$\bar{x} = 11.6$ (from the sample data)
$\sigma = 1.57$ (known from previous experience)
$\mu_0 = 10.0$ (under H_0).

6. $\begin{aligned} T_{1C} &= (11.16 - 10.0)/(1.57/\sqrt{11}) \\ &= 1.16/0.47 \\ &= 2.45. \end{aligned}$

7. From tables of the standard normal distribution (Table A1) $Z(0.025) = 1.96$ and $Z(0.005) = 2.58$. Clearly $|T_{1C}| > Z(0.025)$ since $2.45 > 1.96$, but $|T_{1C}| < Z(0.005)$ since $2.45 < 2.58$. Thus the test is significant at the 5% level. Reject H_0 that the true mean clotting time is 10 min, $0.01 < P < 0.05$.

σ^2 unknown

5. Consider

$$T_2 = (\bar{x} - \mu_0)/(s/\sqrt{n})$$

where

$n = 11$
$\bar{x} = 11.16$ (from the sample data)
$s = 1.99$ (from the sample data)
$\mu_0 = 10.0$ (under H_0).

6. $\begin{aligned} T_{2C} &= (11.16 - 10.0)/(1.99/\sqrt{11}) \\ &= 1.16/0.60 \\ &= 1.93. \end{aligned}$

7. From tables of the t-distribution (Table A3), $t_{10}(0.025) = 2.23$. Hence $|T_{2C}| < t_{10}(0.025)$ since $1.93 < 2.23$. Thus do not reject H_0 that the true mean clotting time is 10 min, $P > 0.05$.

Hypothesis test of a population proportion, π

Consider the experimental situation described in the Example section of Chapter 6 (95% confidence interval for π). π is the true proportion of mites infected after being placed on a cotton rat with microfilarial infection.

1. H_0: $\pi = 0.5$.

2. H_1: $\pi \neq 0.5$, say.

3. A random sample of 50 mites is taken. They are dissected and 10 are found to be infected.

4. No illustration.

5. Consider

$$T_3 = [|p-\pi_0|-1/(2n)]/\sqrt{\pi_0(1-\pi_0)/n}$$

where

$$p = 10/50 = 0.2 \text{ is the sample estimate of } \pi$$
$$\pi_0 = 0.5 \text{ (under } H_0\text{)}$$
$$n = 50.$$

6.
$$\begin{aligned}
T_{3C} &= (|0.2-0.5|-0.01)/\sqrt{(0.5)(1-0.5)/50} \\
&= (0.29)/\sqrt{0.005} \\
&= 4.10.
\end{aligned}$$

7. From tables of the standard normal distribution (Table A1), $Z(0.001) = 3.09$. Hence $|T_{3C}| > Z(0.001)$ since $4.10 > 3.09$. Thus the test is significant at the 0.2% level. Reject H_0 that $\pi = 0.5$ (that the mites are as likely to get infected as not get infected), $P < 0.002$.

Chapter 8
Comparison of Two Means and Two Variances

Introduction

Advances in medicine are effected by new forms of treatment which are adopted if they are of benefit when no alternatives exist or if they are superior to existing treatments. Comparative assessment is thus an integral part of treatment evaluation. The simplest comparative situation is that which concerns the value of a variable in two populations; e.g. the response variable in one population of individuals receiving a new treatment and in another population receiving a control. It is often of interest to determine whether these populations differ from one another with respect to certain characteristics which summarise the values of the variable, such as their means or variances. The techniques of statistical inference provide a solution to the problem. Tests of hypotheses are described which follow the general procedure outlined in Chapter 7.

Assumptions

The variable of interest, x, is assumed to be *normally* distributed in each population. The assumption of normality is not crucial when comparing two means [because of the near normality of the distribution of the sample mean (see p. 41)] but it is important when comparing two variances. The mean and variance of the variable in the ith population ($i = 1, 2$) are μ_i and σ_i^2, respectively.

Sample selection

A test is performed by selecting a random sample of n_i observations from population i ($i = 1, 2$). Two situations are distinguished; when the samples are: (i) *independent:* an individual in one sample is unrelated to any particular individual in the other sample; and (ii) *not independent:* every individual in one sample is paired with an individual in the other sample.

Tests

The tests described in detail are for the equality of:

1. *Two population means* $(H_0: \mu_1 = \mu_2)$
  a. For independent samples when
    (i) variances known,
    (ii) variances unknown but,
      (*A*) variances assumed equal (2 sample *t*-test),
      (*B*) variances assumed unequal and,
        (1) samples small,
        (2) samples large.
  b. For dependent samples (matched pairs) when variances unknown (paired *t*-test).

2. *Two population variances* $(H_0: \sigma_1^2 = \sigma_2^2)$

The test for the equality of two proportions using two independent samples is not discussed in this chapter although a procedure may be adopted for it analogous to the test of equality of two means. Instead, an alternative method (producing identical results) of testing the equivalence of two proportions (the χ^2 test) is described in Chapter 10.

Consideration is also given to testing more than two means and more than two variances.

Hypothesis test: equality of two population means (μ_1, μ_2)

Independent samples

1. Specify $H_0: \mu_1 = \mu_2$ or $\mu_1 - \mu_2 = 0$.
2. Specify $H_1: \mu_1 \neq \mu_2$, say.
3. Select two independent random samples of observations, the set $x_{11}, x_{12}, \ldots, x_{1n_1}$ from population 1 and the set $x_{21}, x_{22}, \ldots, x_{2n_2}$ from population 2. In practice, this is achieved by selecting a sample of individuals and randomly assigning one treatment to n_1 of them and the other treatment to the remaining n_2 individuals.
4. Plot these sample values, most easily using the same scale of measurement for each sample, as shown in Fig. 8.1. The distributions of the observations in both samples should be approximately normal in order that the remaining steps be valid.

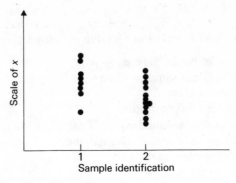

Fig. 8.1   Plot of sample observations (hypothetical) for H_0: $\mu_1 = \mu_2$ (independent samples).

Variances (σ_1^2, σ_2^2) known

5. Consider the test statistic

$$T_4 = (\bar{x}_1 - \bar{x}_2)/\sqrt{\sigma_1^2/n_1 + \sigma_2^2/n_2}$$

where

$$\bar{x}_1 = \sum^{n_1} x_{1j}/n_1 \quad \text{and} \quad \bar{x}_2 = \sum^{n_2} x_{2j}/n_2.$$

This test statistic has an approximately standard normal distribution and is chosen because:

a. A population mean is estimated by a sample mean. The difference between two population means, $\mu_1 - \mu_2$, is estimated by the corresponding difference in their sample means, $\bar{x}_1 - \bar{x}_2$.

b. The sampling distribution of $\bar{x}_i$ is $N(\mu_i, \sigma_i^2/n_i)$ ($i = 1, 2$). Hence, the sampling distribution of $\bar{x}_1 - \bar{x}_2$ is $N(\mu_1 - \mu_2, \sigma_1^2/n_1 + \sigma_2^2/n_2)$. See sampling distribution of a difference in Chapter 5.

c. The sampling distribution of

$$[(\bar{x}_1 - \bar{x}_2) - (\mu_1 - \mu_2)]/\sqrt{\sigma_1^2/n_1 + \sigma_2^2/n_2}$$

is $N(0, 1)$ which has tabulated percentage points.

d. The parameter specification of H_0 is $\mu_1 - \mu_2 = 0$.

6. Compute the value, T_{4C}, of the test statistic from the sample data.

7. Determine the critical region from tables of the standard normal distribution (Table A1). For a two-tailed test at the $200\alpha\%$ level of significance, reject H_0 if $|T_{4C}| > Z(\alpha)$ [i.e. $T_{4C} > Z(\alpha)$ or $T_{4C} < -Z(\alpha)$], $P < 2\alpha$. Do not reject H_0 otherwise, $P > 2\alpha$. In particular $Z(0.025) = 1.96$ for a test at the 5% level of significance.

Variances (σ_1^2, σ_2^2) unknown

Two situations, distinguished by the variances being equal or unequal, are considered. In both cases, steps 1–4 are those described for the test when σ_1^2 and σ_2^2 are known.

VARIANCES EQUAL ($\sigma_1^2 = \sigma_2^2 = \sigma^2$, SAY) (TWO SAMPLE T-TEST)

It is assumed and can be 'confirmed' by a test for homogeneity of variance (Chapter 8) that the variances σ_1^2 and σ_2^2 are equal, their value being an unknown quantity σ^2. The variances estimated from the sample data by

$$s_1^2 = \sum_{}^{n_1}(x_{1j}-\bar{x}_1)^2/(n_1-1) \quad \text{and} \quad s_2^2 = \sum_{}^{n_2}(x_{2j}-\bar{x}_2)^2/(n_2-1)$$

can be *pooled* as a weighted average [the weights are (n_1-1) and (n_2-1)] to estimate σ^2 by

$$s^2 = [(n_1-1)s_1^2+(n_2-1)s_2^2]/(n_1+n_2-2).$$

5. Consider the test statistic

$$T_5 = (\bar{x}_1-\bar{x}_2)/\sqrt{s^2(1/n_1+1/n_2)}$$

whose sampling distribution is t on n_1+n_2-2 degrees of freedom. This test statistic is a logical modification of the test statistic T_4 in which σ_1^2 and σ_2^2 are known, and is obtained by replacing the assumed equal values of σ_1^2 and σ_2^2 by their pooled estimate s^2. The effect is to change the sampling distribution of the test statistic from standard normal to t.

6. Compute the value, T_{5C}, of the test statistic from the sample data.

7. Determine the critical region from tables of the t-distribution (Table A3). For a two-tailed test at the $200\alpha\%$ level of significance reject H_0 if $|T_{5C}| > t_{n_1+n_2-2}(\alpha)$, $P < 2\alpha$. Do not reject H_0 otherwise, $P > 2\alpha$.

This test is called the *two sample t-test*.

VARIANCES UNEQUAL ($\sigma_1^2 \neq \sigma_2^2$)

If the population variances are unequal, then they are estimated *separately* by their respective estimated (sample) variances

$$s_1^2 = \sum^{n_1}(x_{1j}-\bar{x}_1)^2/(n_1-1) \quad \text{and} \quad s_2^2 = \sum^{n_2}(x_{2j}-\bar{x}_2)^2/(n_2-1).$$

Steps **1–4** are those described for the test when σ_1^2 and σ_2^2 are known. Then:

5. Consider the test statistic

$$T_6 = (\bar{x}_1-\bar{x}_2)/\sqrt{s_1^2/n_1+s_2^2/n_2}.$$

The determination of the distribution of this test statistic depends on the sample sizes, n_1 and n_2.

a. n_1 *or* n_2 *small (either* n_1 *or* $n_2 < 20$, *say*)

If n_1 or n_2 is small, then the sampling distribution of T_6 is complex. The reader is referred to the solution of the problem suggested by Behrens, tabulated as Table VI in Fisher, R. A., and Yates, F. (1963), and should not proceed to step **7**. Alternatively, a Wilcoxon rank sum test (see Chapter 12) may be performed.

b. n_1 *and* n_2 *large (both* n_1 *and* $n_2 \geqslant 20$, *say*)

If n_1 and n_2 are large, then T_6 has a distribution which is approximately standard normal. Steps **6** and **7** refer to this situation.

6. Compute the value, T_{6C}, of the test statistic from the sample data.

7. Determine the critical region from tables of the standard normal distribution (Table A1). For a two-tailed test at the $200\alpha\%$ level of significance, reject H_0 if $|T_{6C}| > Z(\alpha)$, $P < 2\alpha$. Do not reject H_0 otherwise, $P > 2\alpha$.

The procedure for testing H_0: $\mu_1 = \mu_2$ is summarised in the flowchart of Fig. 8.2.

Dependent samples (matched pairs)

The random samples are each of size n, and the individual members of one sample are paired with particular members of the other sample. These pairings may consist of: (i) matched individuals in that each pair comprises two individuals who are alike with respect

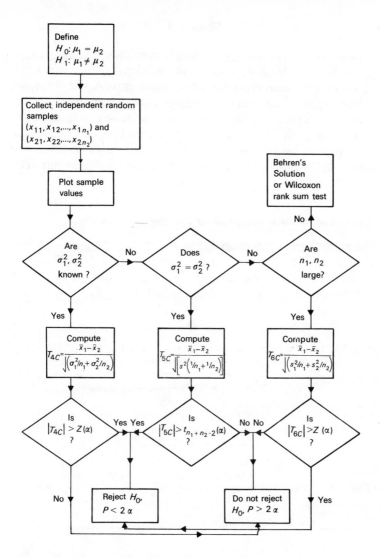

Fig. 8.2 Flow chart of procedure for testing H_0: $\mu_1 = \mu_2$ against H_1: $\mu_1 \neq \mu_2$, when x_i dist. $N(\mu_i, \sigma_i^2)$ $(i = 1, 2)$ independent samples.

$$\bar{x}_i = \sum_{j}^{n_i} x_{ij}/n_i$$

$$s_i^2 = \sum_{j}^{n_i} (x_{ij} - \bar{x}_i)^2/(n_i - 1)$$

$$s^2 = \frac{(n_1 - 1)s_1^2 + (n_2 - 1)s_2^2}{n_1 + n_2 - 2}.$$

to those variables thought to influence response, e.g. age, sex; or (ii) the same individual on different occasions.

A common *example* is when two treatments, A and B say, are to be compared and each patient receives both treatments. Rather than all patients being allocated treatment A (say) before B, and thus possibly introducing an 'order' related bias into the design, some patients receive A before B, and the remainder receive B before A, the order of allocation being determined randomly. This is an example of a *cross-over* design.

Distinction between independent and dependent samples

The paired sample situation differs in design and hence in analysis from that in which there are two independent samples. The information relating to the pairings is retained by considering the difference $d_j = x_{1j} - x_{2j}$ for the jth individual ($j = 1, 2, \ldots, n$), these differences being independent (see Table 8.1).

Table 8.1 Data for paired samples

Individual	Sample 1	Sample 2	Difference $d_j = x_{1j} - x_{2j}$
1	x_{11}	x_{21}	d_1
2	x_{12}	x_{22}	d_2
$\vdots$	$\vdots$	$\vdots$	$\vdots$
n	x_{1n}	x_{2n}	d_n
Total	$\sum x_{1j}$	$\sum x_{2j}$	$\sum_{}^{n} d_j$
Mean	$\bar{x}_1$	$\bar{x}_2$	$\bar{d} = \sum d_j/n$
Estimated variance			$s_d^2 = \sum (d_j - \bar{d})^2/(n-1)$

The sample mean of these differences, $\bar{d} = \sum d_j/n$, is an unbiased estimator of the true population mean of the differences, δ. Also the sample mean of the differences is equal to the difference in the sample means, $\bar{x}_1 - \bar{x}_2$ ($\bar{d} = \sum d_j/n = \sum (x_{1j} - x_{2j})/n = \sum x_{1j}/n - \sum x_{2j}/n = \bar{x}_1 - \bar{x}_2$), which is an unbiased estimator of the difference in the population means, $\mu_1 - \mu_2$. Thus the test H_0: $\mu_1 - \mu_2 = 0$ is equivalent to the test H_0: $\delta = 0$, which is a single sample test of hypothesis concerning a population mean and is described in Chapter 7.

In summary: The test for the equality of two means based on paired samples reduces to a single sample test of the difference from zero of the mean of a set of differences.

Procedure (paired *t*-test)

1. Specify H_0: $\mu_1 = \mu_2$ or $\mu_1 - \mu_2 = 0$ or $\delta = 0$.
2. Specify H_1: $\mu_1 \neq \mu_2$ or $\delta \neq 0$, say.
3. Select two random samples of observations, the set x_{11}, x_{12}, . . . , x_{1n} from population 1 and the set of x_{21}, x_{22}, . . . , x_{2n} from population 2. The observations x_{1j} and x_{2j} ($j = 1, 2, \ldots, n$) are from a matched pair.
4. Plot these sample values, most easily using the same scale of measurement for each sample. Retain the basic information by joining the two observations in each pair by a straight line, as shown in Fig. 8.3. If most of the lines slope upwards (downwards) then it may be expected that the populations have different means. If there is no general tendency for the lines to slope in any one direction then it is unlikely that the means differ.

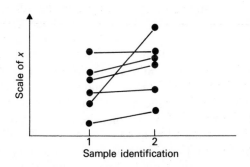

Fig. 8.3 Plot of sample observations (hypothetical) for H_0: $\mu_1 = \mu_2$ (matched pairs).

5. Consider the test statistic

$$T_7 = \bar{d} / \sqrt{s_d^2/n}$$

where the set of differences $d_j = x_{1j} - x_{2j}$ ($j = 1, 2, \ldots, n$) has sample mean $\bar{d} = \sum d_j/n$ and estimated (sample) variance $s_d^2 = \sum (d_j - \bar{d})^2/(n-1)$. It is assumed here, as is generally so, that the true variance of the differences in the population, σ_d^2, is unknown, and it is therefore estimated by s_d^2. The test statistic, T_7, has a t-distribution on $n-1$ degrees of freedom. It is chosen for the reasons similar to those given in Chapter 7 in the description of the procedure for testing H_0: $\mu = \mu_0$. In the present context, $\mu = \delta$ and $\mu_0 = 0$.

6. Compute the value, T_{7C}, of the test statistic from the sample data.

7. Determine the critical region from the tables of the t-distribution (Table A3). For a two-tailed test at the $200\alpha\%$ level of significance, reject H_0 if $|T_{7C}| > t_{n-1}(\alpha)$, $P < 2\alpha$. Do not reject H_0 otherwise, $P > 2\alpha$.

This test is called the *paired t-test*.

Comparison of more than two means

There are various approaches to the problem of comparing the means of more than two groups. All should be considered cautiously and with reservation. This is a complex area although seemingly simple solutions are at hand.

One obvious analysis of the data is achieved by performing t-tests between all possible pairs of means. Each such t-test is a test of a hypothesis of the form $\mu_1 = \mu_2$ or $\mu_1 = \mu_3$, etc. For k groups, there are $\frac{1}{2}k(k-1)$ pairs of means which could be compared and it may be difficult to interpret the results of all these tests. For example, it is quite common to find that the means of groups 1 and 3 do not differ significantly (at the 5% level, say), neither do those of groups 2 and 3, but that the mean of group 1 differs significantly from that of group 3. Part of the difficulty is due to the fact that some of the differences are interrelated [for example, $\mu_3 - \mu_1 = (\mu_3 - \mu_2) + (\mu_2 - \mu_1)$] and part is due to the fact that the more tests that are performed the greater the probability that one of them will produce a significant difference even though the true difference is zero. Clearly, the above-mentioned procedure is not satisfactory. An alternative approach which avoids either '*dredging*' the data (by indiscriminately applying significance tests in the hope that one or more significant differences might appear) or data '*snooping*' (by inspecting the results and then testing those pairs of groups whose means are likely to differ) is advocated.

Rather than test the separate hypotheses $\mu_1 = \mu_2$, $\mu_1 = \mu_3$, etc., it is better *first* to test the overall hypothesis that $\mu_1 = \mu_2 =$

... $= \mu_k$. This is done by performing a one-way analysis of variance (see Chapter 9). If this initial analysis demonstrates a significant difference between groups (giving an indication that at least two groups differ from one another with respect to their means but not indicating which groups they are), the *subsequent examination* is restricted to an analysis of the differences between pairs of groups, selected in advance, which are of logical and/or experimental interest. The difference between the means of any two selected groups is investigated by performing a two sample *t*-test (see pp. 73–74). For each *t*-test, the residual mean square, s_w^2 [which is an estimate of the common population variance and is obtained from the analysis of variance (see pp. 96–97)], is generally used in the denominator of the test statistic, producing a modified test statistic

$$T'_5 = \frac{\bar{x}_1 - \bar{x}_2}{\sqrt{[s_w^2(1/n_1 + 1/n_2)]}}$$

whose sampling distribution is *t* with $N-k$ degrees of freedom (i.e., the degrees of freedom associated with s_w^2). The use of s_w^2 is particularly advantageous when n_1 and n_2 are small.

However, it must be remembered that there are situations in which the structure of the investigation does not lead naturally to the selection of pairs of groups for comparison. Various multiple comparison methods (such as those due to Newman–Keuls and Scheffé) are advocated in such circumstances. These are procedures aimed at reducing the chances of erroneously reporting a number of significant comparisons when the data are dredged. The reader is referred to Armitage, P. (1987) pp. 200–205 for details.

Finally, it should be noted that the methods discussed are only useful when applied to unstructured means. Other techniques can be much better when there is, for example, an increasing stimulus level or some kind of factorial structure.

Hypothesis tests: equality of two population variances (σ_1^2, σ_2^2)

Occasionally it is of interest to investigate evidence of inequality of the variances of two or more populations because: (i) it is of intrinsic importance in the evaluation of the nature of the distributions in the populations; or (ii) it is assumed in tests of hypotheses relating to parameters other than the variance (e.g. the two sample *t*-test for the equality of two means) that the variances are not different. This assumption must be validated.

Procedure (variance ratio test)

1. Specify H_0: $\sigma_1^2 = \sigma_2^2$.
2. Specify H_1: $\sigma_1^2 \neq \sigma_2^2$, say.
3. Select two independent random samples of observations, the set $x_{11}, x_{12}, \ldots, x_{1n_1}$ from population 1 and the set $x_{21}, x_{22}, \ldots, x_{2n_2}$ from population 2.
4. Plot these sample values, most easily using the same scale of measurement for each sample, as shown in Fig. 8.1. The observations from each sample should be approximately normally distributed for the remaining steps to be valid. The assumption of normality is particularly important in the test for the equality of variances.
5. Consider the test statistic

$$T_8 = s_1^2/s_2^2$$

where

$$s_1^2 = \sum_{}^{n_1}(x_{1j}-\bar{x}_1)^2/(n_1-1)$$

and

$$s_2^2 = \sum_{}^{n_2}(x_{2j}-\bar{x}_2)^2/(n_1-1)$$

and

$$s_1^2 \geq s_2^2$$

According to its definition, this ratio is greater than or equal to 1. T_8 has an *F*-distribution on $v_1 = n_1-1$ and $v_2 = n_2-1$ degrees of freedom and is chosen because:

    a. s_1^2 and s_2^2 are the sample statistics which estimate σ_1^2 and σ_2^2.
    b. If *x* is distributed normally in both populations then

$$s_1^2 \text{ dist. } \sigma_1^2\chi_{n_1-1}^2/(n_1-1)$$
$$s_2^2 \text{ dist. } \sigma_2^2\chi_{n_2-1}^2/(n_2-1)$$

(see Chapter 5).

c. Thus

$$u = (n_1-1)s_1^2/\sigma_1^2 \text{ dist. } \chi_{n_1-1}^2$$
$$v = (n_2-1)s_2^2/\sigma_2^2 \text{ dist. } \chi_{n_2-1}^2,$$

independently, so

$$\left(\frac{u}{n_1-1}\right)\Big/\left(\frac{v}{n_2-1}\right) = \left(\frac{s_1^2}{\sigma_1^2}\right)\Big/\left(\frac{s_2^2}{\sigma_2^2}\right) \text{ dist. } F_{n_1-1,\, n_2-1}$$

(see Chapter 5) which has tabulated percentage points.

   d. The parameter specification of H_0 is $\sigma_1^2 = \sigma_2^2$.

6. Compute the value, T_{8C}, of the test statistic from the sample data.

7. Determine the critical region from tables of the F-distribution (Table A4). For a two-tailed test at the $200\alpha\%$ level of significance, reject H_0 if $T_{8C} > F_{n_1-1,\, n_2-1}(\alpha)$, $P < 2\alpha$. Do not reject H_0 otherwise, $P > 2\alpha$.

   Note: Although a two-tailed test of significance is described, only the upper tail of the F-distribution need be considered. This is a consequence of defining the variance ratio as the larger estimated variance divided by the smaller. This technique can be shown to be equivalent to the alternative approach of not placing a restriction on the variance ratio and considering both tails of the F-distribution.

Comparison of more than two variances

Occasionally (see p. 96) it is of interest to investigate evidence of inequality of more than two population variances. In particular, the analysis of variance techniques described in Chapter 9 make an assumption of *homoscedasticity* (equal variances, see p. 103) and this assumption may need to be validated. It should be noted that the F-test in the analysis of variance is quite insensitive to heterogeneity of variance when the number of observations in each group are equal. Furthermore, tests of homoscedasticity are generally sensitive to non-normality of the data, and, in any case, often do not produce a significant result even when the true variances differ. Thus a formal test of homoscedasticity is not employed very often and is not discussed in depth in this text. However, should the need for a test of homoscedasticity arise, one of the approximate tests (each based on the assumption that the observations are randomly selected from normally distributed data) mentioned below may be used. Both tests are discussed in Pearson, E. S. and Hartley, H. O. (1966). The approximate tests of homoscedasticity are:

1. *Bartlett's test* based on a modification of the likelihood ratio statistic. Table 32 of Pearson and Hartley's book (1966) provides 5% and 1% percentage points for the relevant M statistic.
2. A test based on the ratio of the largest to the smallest estimates of variance. Table 31 of Pearson and Hartley's book (1966) provides 5% and 1% percentage points for this ratio.

The computation involved in Bartlett's test is often heavy. For this reason, the second test may be preferred. It provides a quick assessment of heterogeneity of variance when the number of observations in each sample are equal (when the numbers differ, an approximate procedure is to use their average in the table).

Confidence intervals in relation to hypothesis tests

The function of confidence intervals extends beyond providing limits for estimators of unknown population parameters and into the realms of hypothesis testing.

1. A confidence interval may be used to *test* an hypothesis. In general terms, the null hypothesis H_0: $P = P_0$, where P is any parameter and P_0 a particular value (e.g. H_0: $\mu = \mu_0$ or H_0: $\mu_1 - \mu_2 = 0$), is rejected at the $200\alpha\%$ level of significance if P_0 lies outside the $100(1-2\alpha)\%$ confidence interval for P, and not rejected otherwise.

Proof (by example)
    Suppose

$$x \text{ dist. } N(\mu, \sigma^2)$$

Consider

$$H_0: \mu = \mu_0$$
$$H_1: \mu \neq \mu_0, \text{ say.}$$

The test statistic is $T_1 = (\bar{x} - \mu_0)/(\sigma/\sqrt{n})$ which has a standard normal distribution (see Chapter 7). H_0 is rejected at the $200\alpha\%$ level of significance if the value, T_{1C}, of the test statistic computed from the sample falls in the critical region. The critical region is the set of values of the test statistic greater than $Z(\alpha)$ and less than $-Z(\alpha)$ (e.g. if $2\alpha = 0.05$, $Z(\alpha) = 1.96$).

But if

$$\frac{\bar{x}-\mu_0}{\sigma/\sqrt{n}} > Z(\alpha)$$

then

$$\mu_0 < \bar{x}-Z(\alpha)\frac{\sigma}{\sqrt{n}}$$

and if

$$\frac{\bar{x}-\mu_0}{\sigma/\sqrt{n}} < -Z(\alpha)$$

then

$$\mu_0 > \bar{x}+Z(\alpha)\frac{\sigma}{\sqrt{n}}.$$

Hence H_0 is rejected if μ_0 lies outside the interval

$$[\bar{x}-Z(\alpha)\sigma/\sqrt{n}, \bar{x}+Z(\alpha)\sigma/\sqrt{n}].$$

This interval is the $100(1-2\alpha)\%$ confidence interval for μ.

2. In addition to providing a test for an hypothesis, a confidence interval also provides an *interval estimate* for the parameter under test. Thus the confidence interval approach to hypothesis testing detracts from the well-defined decision to reject or not reject H_0 on the basis of fairly arbitrary criteria (e.g. the choice of significance level) and encourages an evaluation of the situation by consideration of the estimated magnitude of the effects. In particular, the confidence intervals summarised in Table 8.2 may be found to be useful in relation to the tests of hypotheses mentioned in Chapters 7 and 8.

Examples

Equality of two population means

Independent samples

Interest is centred on the difference between the distributions of

Table 8.2 Confidence intervals for various parameters

	Parameter	Conditions	$100(1-2\alpha)\%$ confidence interval
Single sample	Mean (μ)	(i) σ^2 known	$\bar{x} \pm Z(\alpha)\sigma/\sqrt{n}$
		(ii) σ^2 unknown	$\bar{x} \pm t_{n-1}(\alpha)s/\sqrt{n}$
	Proportion (π)	Large sample	$*p \pm Z(\alpha)\sqrt{p(1-p)/n}$
Two independent samples	Difference in means $(\mu_1 - \mu_2)$	(i) σ_1^2, σ_2^2 known	$(\bar{x}_1 - \bar{x}_2) \pm Z(\alpha)\sqrt{\dfrac{\sigma_1^2}{n_1} + \dfrac{\sigma_2^2}{n_2}}$
		(ii) $\sigma_1^2 = \sigma_2^2$ unknown	$(\bar{x}_1 - \bar{x}_2) \pm t_{n_1+n_2-2}(\alpha)\sqrt{s^2\left(\dfrac{1}{n_1} + \dfrac{1}{n_2}\right)}$
		(iii) $\sigma_1^2 \neq \sigma_2^2$ unknown large samples	$(\bar{x}_1 - \bar{x}_2) \pm Z(\alpha)\sqrt{\dfrac{s_1^2}{n_1} + \dfrac{s_2^2}{n_2}}$
	Difference in proportions $(\pi_1 - \pi_2)$	Large samples	$\dagger(p_1 - p_2) \pm Z(\alpha)\sqrt{\dfrac{p_1(1-p_1)}{n_1} + \dfrac{p_2(1-p_2)}{n_2}}$
Matched pairs	Difference in means $(\mu_1 - \mu_2)$	σ_d^2 unknown	$\bar{d} \pm t_{n-1}(\alpha)s_d/\sqrt{n}$

Single sample: x dist. $N(\mu, \sigma^2)$, $\bar{x} = \sum x_i/n$, $s^2 = \sum(x_i - \bar{x})^2/(n-1)$.

Two samples $(i = 1, 2)$: x_i dist. $N(\mu_i, \sigma_i^2)$, $\bar{x}_i = \sum_{i}^{n_i} x_{ij}/n_i$, $s_i^2 = \sum_{j}^{n_i}(x_{ij} - \bar{x}_i)^2/(n_i - 1)$,

$s^2 = [(n_1 - 1)s_1^2 + (n_2 - 1)s_2^2]/(n_1 + n_2 - 2)$.

Matched pairs: $d_j = x_{1j} - x_{2j}$, $\bar{d} = \sum_{}^{n} d_j/n$, $s_d^2 = \sum_{}^{n}(d_j - \bar{d})^2/(n-1)$.

*The continuity correction $1/(2n)$ may be applied. †The continuity correction $(n_1 + n_2)/(2n_1 n_2)$ may be applied.

the age at onset of symptoms in males and females suffering from lung cancer. The mean and variance of the distribution in female patients are μ_1 and σ_1^2, respectively; in male patients these parameters are μ_2 and σ_2^2.

1. H_0: $\mu_1 = \mu_2$.
2. H_1: $\mu_1 \neq \mu_2$.
3. The ages at onset of symptoms shown in Table E8.1 were recorded in a random sample of 12 female lung cancer patients and in an independent random sample of 13 male lung cancer patients.

Table E8.1 Age (years) at onset of symptoms in a sample of male cancer patients and in an independent sample of female cancer patients

Females	58	52	50	49	56	52	54	48	41	37	67	70	
Males	26	41	57	66	36	55	41	61	53	50	52	37	50

Source: Hypothetical data.

From Table E5.1:

Females	Males
$n_1 = 12$	$n_2 = 13$
$\sum_1 x = 634$	$\sum_2 x = 625$
$\bar{x}_1 = 634/12 = 52.83$	$\bar{x}_2 = 625/13 = 48.08$
$\sum(x - \bar{x}_1)^2 = 971.68$	$\sum(x - \bar{x}_2)^2 = 1518.92$
$s_1^2 = 971.68/11 = 88.33.$	$s_2^2 = 1518.92/12 = 126.58.$

4. The sample values are plotted in Fig. E8.1. It would appear, from inspection by eye of Fig. E8.1, that there is no difference between the means, and that the ages in each sample are approximately normally distributed.

VARIANCES (σ_1^2, σ_2^2) KNOWN (VERY UNLIKELY)

5. Consider

$$T_4 = \frac{\bar{x}_1 - \bar{x}_2}{\sqrt{(\sigma_1^2/n_1 + \sigma_2^2/n_2)}}$$

where

$$\bar{x}_1 = 52.83, \ \bar{x}_2 = 48.08$$
$$\sigma_1^2 = 93 \ \text{(prior knowledge)}$$
$$\sigma_2^2 = 120 \ \text{(prior knowledge)}$$
$$n_1 = 12, \ n_2 = 13.$$

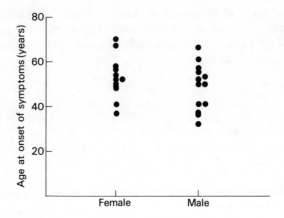

Fig. E8.1 Ages (years) at onset of symptoms in males and females. Source: Table E8.1.

6.
$$T_{4C} = (52.83-48.08)/\sqrt{(93/12)+(120/13)}$$
$$= 4.75/\sqrt{16.98}$$
$$= (4.75)/(4.12)$$
$$= 1.15.$$

7. From tables of the standard distribution (Table A1), $Z(0.025) = 1.96$. Hence $|T_{4C}| < Z(0.025)$ since $1.15 < 1.96$. Thus do not reject H_0 that there is no difference in the mean age at onset of symptoms between females and males suffering from lung cancer, $P > 0.05$.

Furthermore, the 95% confidence limits for the difference in the true means ($\mu_1-\mu_2$, estimated by 4.75 years) are:

$$(\bar{x}_1-\bar{x}_2)\pm1.96\sqrt{\sigma_1^2/n_1+\sigma_2^2/n_2} = 4.75\pm1.96\,(4.12)$$
$$= 4.75\pm8.076$$
$$= -3.33 \text{ and } 12.83 \text{ years.}$$

VARIANCES (σ_1^2, σ_2^2) UNKNOWN (MORE LIKELY)

5. It is assumed (see below: the F-test) that the variances σ_1^2 and σ_2^2 are equal and each can be equated to σ^2. The estimated variances $s_1^2 = 88.33$ and $s_2^2 = 126.58$ are pooled to estimate σ^2 by

$$s^2 = [(n_1-1)s_1^2+(n_2-1)s_2^2]/(n_1+n_2-2)$$
$$= [(11)(88.33)+(12)(126.58)]/(12+13-2)$$
$$= 108.29.$$

Consider

$$T_5 = \frac{\bar{x}_1 - \bar{x}_2}{\sqrt{\left[s^2\left(\dfrac{1}{n_1} + \dfrac{1}{n_2}\right)\right]}}.$$

6.
$$\begin{aligned}
T_{5C} &= (52.83 - 48.08)/\sqrt{(108.29)(1/12 + 1/13)} \\
&= (4.75)/\sqrt{17.35} \\
&= 1.14.
\end{aligned}$$

7. From tables of the *t*-distribution (Table A3), $t_{23}(0.025) = 2.07$. Hence $|T_{5C}| < t_{23}(0.025)$ since $1.14 < 2.07$. Thus do not reject H_0 that there is no difference in the mean age at onset of symptoms between females and males suffering from lung cancer, $P > 0.05$.

Furthermore, the 95% confidence limits for difference in the true means ($\mu_1 - \mu_2$, estimated by 4.75 years) are

$$\begin{aligned}
(\bar{x}_1 - \bar{x}_2) \pm t_{23}(0.025)\sqrt{s^2\left(\frac{1}{n_1} + \frac{1}{n_2}\right)} &= 4.75 \pm 2.069 \ (4.165) \\
&= 4.75 \pm 8.618 \\
&= -3.87 \text{ and } 13.37 \text{ years.}
\end{aligned}$$

Table E8.2 Fibrinogen concentration (mg/100 ml) in 10 patients treated with clofibrate

Patient (i)	Fibrinogen concentration (mg/100 ml)		Difference $d_i = (x_{1i} - x_{2i})$
	Pre-treatment (x_{1i})	Post-treatment (x_{2i})	
1	379	325	54
2	351	333	18
3	420	391	29
4	303	275	28
5	346	311	35
6	370	323	47
7	381	370	11
8	349	354	−5
9	284	249	35
10	380	315	65
Total			317

Source: Dr G.P.M. Crawford (personal communication).

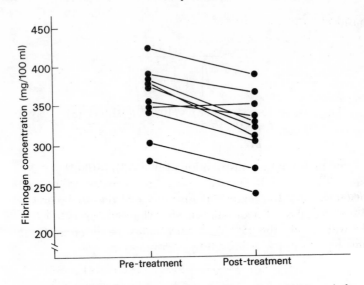

Fig. E8.2 Fibrinogen concentration (mg/100 ml) in patients before and after treatment with clofibrate. Source: Table E8.2.

Dependent samples (paired *t*-test)

It is suggested that patients with ischaemic heart disease should be treated with clofibrate which is believed to lower plasma fibrinogen concentration. It is of interest to determine whether their mean concentration of fibrinogen (mg/100 ml) before treatment (μ_1) is significantly higher than their mean concentration after 8 weeks of treatment (μ_2).

1. H_0: $\mu_1 = \mu_2$.
2. H_1: $\mu_1 > \mu_2$.
3. A random sample of 10 patients with ischaemic heart disease is selected. Each patient has his fibrinogen concentration measured before treatment with clofibrate and 8 weeks after treatment. The results are shown in Table E8.2.
4. The data are plotted in Fig. E8.2. It would appear that for most of the patients, the pre-treatment concentration of fibrinogen is higher than the concentration 8 weeks after treatment. The data values appear to be approximately normally distributed in each sample.
5. Consider

$$T_7 = \bar{d}/\sqrt{s_d^2/n}$$

where

$$\bar{d} = 317/10 = 31.7$$
$$\sum(d-\bar{d})^2 = 3846.1$$
$$s_d^2 = \sum(d-\bar{d})^2/(n-1) = (3846.1)/9 = 427.34.$$

6.

$$T_{7C} = \frac{31.7}{\sqrt{[(427.34)/10]}} = \frac{31.7}{6.54} = 4.85.$$

7. From tables of the t-distribution (Table A3), $t_9(0.0005) = 4.78$. Hence $|T_{7C}| > t_9(0.0005)$ since $4.85 > 4.78$. Thus (using a *one-tailed* test) reject H_0 that there is no difference between the concentration of fibrinogen before treatment with clofibrate and 8 weeks after treatment, $P < 0.0005$. Furthermore, the 95% confidence limits for the true mean difference are

$$\bar{d} \pm t_9(0.025)\sqrt{s_d^2/n} = 31.7 \pm 2.262\ (6.54)$$
$$= 16.91 \text{ and } 46.49 \text{ mg/100 ml.}$$

Comparison of more than two means

Thirty-three patients with hypertrophic cardiomyopathy were studied to determine whether the presence of an intraventricular pressure gradient impaired left ventricular emptying (see Siegel, R. J. and Criley, J. M., 1985, pp. 283–291). The patients were classified into three groups on the basis of the absence of a resting or inducible intraventricular gradient (Group 1), an inducible gradient (Group 2), and a resting gradient of > 25 mm Hg (Group 3). The left ventricular ejection fractions were calculated for each patient after cine-angiography had been performed and their values are presented in Table E8.3 and illustrated in Fig. E8.3.

The result of the F-test from the one-way analysis of variance was significant ($P < 0.001$) (see Examples section in Chapter 9), suggesting that at least two groups may differ from one another with respect to their population means.

As interest was centred on comparing ventricular emptying in patients with and without a pressure gradient, the next stage of the analysis was restricted to two modified t-tests comparing the mean of Group 1 with the means of each of the other two groups. The conventional two-sample t-test was modified by using the residual mean square, $s_w^2 = 57.953$, in the denominator of the test statistic.

Table E8.3 Angiographic left ventricular ejection fractions (%) in 33 patients with hypertrophic cardiomyopathy with no gradient (Group 1), an inducible gradient (Group 2), and a resting gradient (Group 3)

| | Group (i) | | | |
	1	2	3	Total
	59	76	74	
	70	64	87	
	76	89	89	
	76	83	89	
	79	86	90	
	82	89	90	
	84	89	90	
	78	89	94	
		91	96	
		95	98	
			98	
			98	
			99	
			94	
			96	
Sample number, n_i	8	10	15	$N = 33$
Total in i^{th} sample, T_i	604	851	1382	$T = 2837$
Sample mean, $\bar{x}_i = T_i/n_i$	75.5	85.1	92.13˙	
Sample variance, s_i^2	62.286	80.76˙	41.124	

Source: Siegel, R. J. and Criley, J. M. (1985) Comparison of ventricular emptying with and without a pressure gradient in patients with hypertrophic cardiomyopathy. *Br. Heart J.*, **53**, 283–291.

Group 1 versus Group 2

$$T_5' = \frac{\bar{x}_2 - \bar{x}_1}{\sqrt{[s_w^2(1/n_1 + 1/n_2)]}}$$

$$T_{5C}' = \frac{85.1 - 75.5}{\sqrt{[57.953(1/8 + 1/10)]}} = 2.66.$$

From the table of the t-distribution (Table A3), using $33 - 3 = 30$ degrees of freedom, $t_{30}(0.025) = 2.042$ and $t_{30}(0.005) = 2.750$. Hence $0.01 < P < 0.05$.

Furthermore, 95% confidence limits for the difference in the

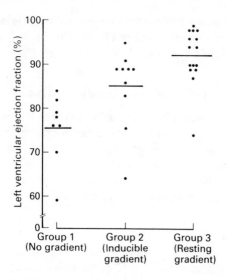

Fig. E8.3 Angiographic left ventricular ejection fractions in three groups of patients with hypertrophic cardiomyopathy.

true means (estimated by $85.1 - 75.5 = 9.6\%$) are given by

$$(\bar{x}_2 - \bar{x}_1) \pm t_{30}(0.025) \ \sqrt{s_w^2(1/n_1 + 1/n_2)}$$
$$= (85.1 - 75.5) \pm 2.042 \ \sqrt{57.953(1/8 + 1/10)}$$
$$= 9.6 \pm 7.3736$$
$$= 2.23\% \text{ and } 16.97\%$$

Group 1 versus Group 3

$$T_5'' = \frac{\bar{x}_3 - \bar{x}_1}{\sqrt{[s_w^2(1/n_1 + 1/n_3)]}}$$
$$T_{5C}'' = \frac{92.13 - 75.5}{\sqrt{[57.953(1/8 + 1/15)]}} = 4.99$$

From the table of the t-distribution, $t_{30}(0.0005) = 3.819$. Hence $P < 0.001$.

Furthermore, the 95% confidence limits for the difference in the true mean (estimated by $92.13 - 75.5 = 16.63\%$) are given by

$$(92.13 - 75.5) \pm 2.042\sqrt{57.953(1/8 + 1/15)} = 16.63 \pm 6.8056$$
$$= 9.83\% \text{ and } 23.44\%.$$

Thus, the mean left ventricular ejection fraction was significantly higher in Group 2 than in Group 1 $(0.01 < P < 0.05)$, and significantly higher in Group 3 than in Group 1 $(P < 0.001)$.

Equality of two population variances

Consider the problem discussed earlier in these Examples in which interest is centred on the difference between the distributions of the age at the onset of symptoms in males and females suffering from lung cancer. The mean and variance of the distribution of the age in female patients are μ_1 and σ_1^2, respectively; in male patients these parameters are μ_2 and σ_2^2.

1. H_0: $\sigma_1^2 = \sigma_2^2$.
2. H_1: $\sigma_1^2 \neq \sigma_2^2$.
3. The ages at onset of symptoms shown in Table E8.1 were recorded in a random sample of 12 female lung cancer patients and in an independent random sample of 13 male lung cancer patients.
4. The sample data are presented visually in Fig. E8.1. It does not appear from the diagram that the spread of the observations in males is different from that in females. The ages at onset of symptoms in each sample appear to be approximately normally distributed.
5. Consider $T_8 = s_1^2/s_2^2 > 1$.
6. In reality, $s_1^2 = 88.33$ (females) and $s_2^2 = 126.58$ (males). To satisfy the condition that the ratio of the estimated variances be greater than one, take

$$T_{8C} = (126.58)/(88.33) = 1.43.$$

7. From tables of the F-distribution (Table A4), $F_{12,11}(0.05) = 2.72$. Hence $T_{8C} < F_{12,11}(0.05)$ since $1.43 < 2.72$. Thus do not reject H_0 that there is no difference between the variances of the distributions of the age at onset of symptoms in males and females suffering from lung cancer, $P > 0.05$.

Confidence intervals in relation to hypothesis tests

Consider the problem discussed in the Examples to Chapters 6 and 7, concerning the clotting time (min) of plasma. A random sample of 11 subjects is selected and the clotting time of plasma of each is measured ($\bar{x} = 11.16$, $s = 1.99$, $n = 11$). The 95% confidence interval for μ, the true mean clotting time of plasma (when

σ^2 is unknown and estimated in the sample by s^2), is the interval 9.82 min to 12.50 min (see Examples section in Chapter 6). Thus to test the null hypothesis that the true mean clotting time, μ, is 10 min (as in Examples section in Chapter 7), observe whether the 95% confidence interval for μ contains the value of μ under H_0, i.e. 10 min. The interval (9.82, 12.50) contains the value 10. Hence do not reject H_0 that the true mean clotting time for plasma is 10 min, $P > 0.05$. This accords with the alternative method of testing H_0 by referring T_{2C} to tables of the t-distribution (see Examples section into Chapter 7).

Chapter 9
Analysis of Variance

This chapter does not attempt to provide a comprehensive account of the analysis of variance but rather serves as an introduction to the general concepts involved. Attention is focused on one-way and two-way analyses of variance as these are the natural extensions, when more than two groups are involved, to the two-sample and paired t-tests discussed in Chapter 8.

General concepts

The analysis of variance is concerned with analysing experimental data to evaluate the contribution of certain factors to the total variation of the variable under study. The total variation exhibited by a set of observations is separated into its constituent parts, one constituent measuring the variability due to unexplained causes or experimental error (the residual), and each of the other constituents being associated with defined sources of variation used as criteria for classifying the observations. All these measures of variation can be tabulated in an analysis of variance table. The contribution of any factor to the total variation of the variable under study is often (depending on the nature of the data) evaluated by comparing its variation with that of the residual, leading to an F-test.

Useful terms

Factor

A quality, or property, defining a set of categories or classes, and seen as a possible cause of variation.

Level

The different categories of a factor are called levels.

Experimental design

The structure or pattern of the experiment, described by the factors appearing in it and the way in which the various factors are combined. The principles of design are discussed briefly on pp. 191–197. The one- and two-way analyses of variance are based on different forms of experimental design.

Block

This is a group of units constructed so that the units within a block are, as far as possible, homogeneous, exhibiting less variation than that between blocks. The *purpose* of blocking is to increase the precision of the relevant treatment comparisons (determined by the intra-block rather than the inter-block variation).

A *randomised block* design is one in which treatments are allocated randomly within blocks of homogeneous units, thus allowing for one extraneous source of variation. A special form of a randomised block design is a *within-patient study* which is particularly useful in medicine when patients often vary in their initial disease state and in their response to therapy. In such a within-patient study, each block comprises one patient, and the order in which that patient receives each treatment is determined randomly (see also within-patient studies, p. 195).

More complex designs incorporate blocking to allow simultaneously for more than one extraneous source of variation (for example, a latin square design, pp. 107–108).

Residual variation

This measures the variability due to unexplained causes or experimental error. It is that part of the variation which remains after the effect of certain systematic elements is removed.

Degrees of freedom

These may be viewed in two ways. (i) The degrees of freedom of a statistic are the number of unrestricted variables associated with it (e.g. the degrees of freedom of $s^2 = \sum_{i=1}^{n} (x_i - \bar{x})^2/(n-1)$, are $n-1$ since the deviations are restricted by the one condition that

$\sum_{i=1}^{n} (x_i - \bar{x}) = 0$). Alternatively, (ii) the degrees of freedom of a statistic are the number of independent observations in the sample minus the number of population parameters which must be estimated from the sample observations in order to define the statistic (e.g. the population mean is estimated by $\bar{x}$ in $s^2 = \sum_{i=1}^{n} (x_i - \bar{x})^2/(n-1)$ so that the degrees of freedom of s^2 are $n-1$).

One-way analysis of variance

The one-way analysis of variance is a form of design and subsequent analysis utilised when the data can be classified into k categories or levels of a single factor, and the equality of the k class means in the population is to be investigated. It is the simplest type of analysis of variance, and is a generalisation of the two-sample t-test in which there are only two classes or groups.

Notation

Suppose the observation, x, on each experimental unit can be classified into one of k categories or groups and that, after sampling, the ith group contains n_i observations. The data are presented in Table 9.1.

Estimates of the population variance, σ^2

1. Between groups. Assuming that the variance of the observations within a group is the same for all groups (see Chapter 8 for a test of homogeneity of variance, pp. 81–82) the separate estimates of variance of the observations within a group, $s_i^2 = \sum_{j=1}^{n_i} (x_{ij} - \bar{x}_i)^2/$ $(n_i - 1)(i = 1, 2, \ldots, k)$, can be pooled (analogous to the procedure in the t-test, p. 73) to estimate the common population variance, σ^2, by the weighted average

$$s_w^2 = \sum_{i=1}^{k} (n_i - 1)s_i^2 \bigg/ \left[\sum_{i=1}^{n} (n_i - 1) \right]$$

$$= \sum_{i=1}^{k} (n_i - 1)s_i^2/(N-k)$$

Table 9.1 Sample of observations in a one-way design

	Group						
	1	2	. . .	i	. . .	k	
	x_{11}	x_{12}	. . .	x_{1i}	. . .	x_{1k}	
	x_{21}	x_{22}		x_{2i}		x_{2k}	
	.	.		.		.	
	.	.		.		.	
	.	.		.		.	
	$x_{n_1 1}$	.		$x_{n_i i}$		.	
		.				.	
		$x_{n_2 2}$				$x_{n_k k}$	
Number of obs. n_i	n_1	n_2		n_i		n_k	$N = \sum\limits_{i=1}^{k} n_i$
Sum of x's	T_1	T_2		T_i		T_k	$T = \sum\limits_{i=1}^{k} T_i$
Sample mean of x's	$\bar{x}_1$	$\bar{x}_2$		$\bar{x}_i$		$\bar{x}_k$	$\bar{x} = T/N$
Estimated variance	s_1^2	s_2^2		s_i^2		s_k^2	

where $T_i = \sum\limits_{j=1}^{n_i} x_{ij}$

$\bar{x}_i = T_i/n_i$

$s_i^2 = \sum\limits_{j=1}^{n_i} (x_{ij} - \bar{x}_i)^2/(n_i - 1)$

with $N-k$ degrees of freedom (i.e. each of the s_i^2 ($i = 1, 2, \ldots, k$) has $n_i - 1$ degrees of freedom so that s_w^2 has $\sum\limits_{i=1}^{k} (n_i - 1) = N - k$ degrees of freedom). s_w^2 is often called the *residual mean square* or the *within group mean square*.

2. Within groups. For simplicity, the derivation of an alternative expression for the estimate of σ^2 is confined to the case in which the number of observations in each group is equal, i.e. $n_i = n (i = 1, 2, \ldots, k)$ Now

a. The variance of the sample mean is $\text{Var}(\bar{x}) = \sigma^2/n$ (see p. 41).

b. Under the null hypothesis that all the group means are equal (their common value, μ, being estimated in the sample by $\sum\limits_{i=1}^{k} \bar{x}_i/k = \sum\limits_{i=1}^{k} T_i/(nk) = T/N = \bar{x}$), the estimated variance of

the sample mean is obtained by applying the usual variance formula to the means rather than to the observations, i.e. it is
$$\sum_{i=1}^{k} (\bar{x}_i - \bar{x})^2/(k-1)$$ with $k-1$ degrees of freedom.
Thus by equating the two expressions for the variance of the sample mean and its estimate from **a** and **b**, it can be seen that, under the null hypothesis, σ^2 is estimated by

$$s_b^2 = n \sum_{i=1}^{k} (\bar{x}_i - \bar{x})^2/(k-1)$$

with $k-1$ degrees of freedom.

Note: It can be shown that, in general [i.e. when the n_i vary $(i = 1, 2, \ldots, k)$], σ^2 is estimated by

$$s_b^2 = \sum_{i=1}^{k} n_i(\bar{x}_i - \bar{x})^2/(k-1).$$

s_b^2 is often called the *between group mean square*.

Ratio of estimated variances

If the true population means of the k groups are equal, s_b^2 and s_w^2 are two estimates of the same underlying quantity, the common population variance, σ^2. Then the ratio s_b^2/s_w^2 is approximately unity. This ratio is greater than one when the k means differ systematically so that s_b^2 is inflated (since it contains a reflection of the between group differences as well as the variability of the observations). In fact, under the null hypothesis that the group means are equal, the ratio s_b^2/s_w^2 has an F-distribution with $v_1 = k-1$ and $v_2 = N-k$ degrees of freedom, provided the observations in the samples are independently and normally distributed (see variance ratio test procedure, pp. 78–81). Thus the ratio s_b^2/s_w^2 is an indicator of homogeneity amongst the group means, and it is used in the formal hypothesis test procedure described below.

Test of hypothesis

(Equality of k population means ($\mu_1, \mu_2, \ldots, \mu_k$) using independent samples)

1. Specify H_0: $\mu_1 = \mu_2 = \ldots = \mu_k = \mu$, say.
2. Specify H_1: $\mu_i(i = 1, 2, \ldots, k)$ are not all equal.

3. Select k independent random samples of observations, the set $(x_{i1}, x_{i2}, \ldots, x_{in_i}; i = 1, 2, \ldots, k)$. Present the data in a table of the form shown in Table 9.1.

4. Plot the sample values using the same scale of measurement for each sample, as shown in Fig. 9.1. The distribution of the observations in every sample should be approximately *normal* and the variability of the observations should be approximately *constant* in all samples in order that the remaining steps be valid.

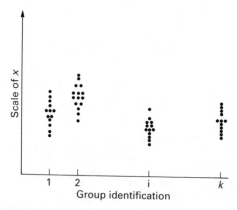

Fig. 9.1 Plot of sample observations (hypothetical) for H_0: $\mu_1 = \mu_2 = \ldots = \mu_k$ (independent samples).

5. Consider the test statistic

$$T_9 = s_b^2/s_w^2,$$

where

$$s_b^2 = \sum_{i=1}^{k} n_i(\bar{x}_i - \bar{x})^2/(k-1)$$

and

$$s_w^2 = \sum_{i=1}^{k} (n_i-1)s_i^2/(N-k)$$

where

$$s_i^2 = \sum_{j=1}^{n_i} (x_{ij}-\bar{x}_i)^2/(n_i-1).$$

This test statistic has an *F*-distribution with $v_1 = k-1$ and $v_2 = N-k$ degrees of freedom.

6. Compute the value, T_{9C}, of the test statistic. It can be computed quite easily using only a calculator (many of which have variance functions), although the analysis of variance is often performed on a computer. In particular, (i) if $n_i = n$ for all i $(i = 1, 2, \ldots, k)$ then s_b^2 is obtained by applying the usual variance formula to the means $\bar{x}_i (i = 1, 2, \ldots, k)$ rather than to the observations, and then multiplying by n. For varying n_i, the following identity may be useful:

$$(k-1)s_b^2 = \sum_{i=1}^{k} T_i^2/n_i - T^2/N.$$

(ii) s_w^2 is a function of s_i^2, and all the s_i^2 can be calculated routinely. Alternatively, it can be shown that

$$(N-k)s_w^2 = \sum_{i}^{k}\sum_{j}^{n_i} x_{ij}^2 - \sum_{i=1}^{k} T_i^2/n_i.$$

where $\sum_{i}^{k}\sum_{j}^{n_i} x_{ij}^2$ is the sum of *all* the x^2's.

7. Determine the critical region from tables of the *F*-distribution (Table A4). Departures from H_0 tend to give values of T_{9C} greater than unity so that a one-tailed test is appropriate. For a one-tailed test at the $100\alpha\%$ level of significance, reject H_0 if $T_{9C} > F_{k-1,N-k}(\alpha)$, $P < \alpha$. Do not reject H_0 otherwise.

Violations of the assumptions in one-way analysis of variance

It is assumed that the observations in each group are normally distributed and that their true variance is constant for all groups.

The *F*-test is a robust test in that it is (i) insensitive to non-normality of the data, and (ii) insensitive to variance inequalities provided the number of observations in each group, n_i, are equal $(i = 1, 2, \ldots, k)$. If the n_i are unequal, variance inequalities (particularly systematic differences) are more serious.

Transformations of the scale of measurement may produce normality of the data and/or homogeneity of variance (see pp. 171–174).

Note: There is a χ^2 test for homogeneity of *k* variances (see pp. 81–82) but this test is as sensitive to non-normality of the data as it is to differences in the variances.

One-way analysis of variance for two groups

When there are only two groups (i.e. $k = 2$), the F-test is equivalent to the two-sample t-test (see pp. 71–73). In particular, it can be shown that $T_9 = T_5^2$, i.e. the test statistic in the one-way analysis of variance is equal to the square of the test-statistic in the two-sample t-test. Furthermore, the significance levels in the F-table (Table A4) with $v_1 = 1$ and $v_2 = N-2$ are equal to the squares of those in the t-table (Table A3) with degrees of freedom $v = v_2 = N-2$.

Although either test can be used, the t-test is generally preferred as it provides information concerning the size and the direction of the difference in the means.

Two-way analysis of variance

The two-way analysis of variance is appropriate when the data are classified simultaneously by two factors such that *each* level of one factor can be combined with *all* levels of the other factor. The levels of the factors are generally represented by the (r, say) rows and (c, say) columns of a two-way table.

Consideration is given here only to the simple situation in which there is *no replication* (i.e. there is only one observation in each cell corresponding to a row and column specification) and there are *no missing observations*. The sample data can then be presented in a table of the form shown in Table 9.2.

Interest is generally centred on the differences between the means of the groups distinguished by the levels of one factor. When one factor designates 'treatments' and is of primary importance, and the other factor consists of randomised blocks of experimental units, the design is a *randomised block* design. In such circumstances, the two-way analysis of variance can be viewed as a generalisation of the paired t-test (pp. 77–78), appropriate for any number of groups.

Alternatively, both factors may be of intrinsic interest which happens with factorial experiments. Then the differences between the means are investigated for each of the two factors.

Table 9.2 Sample of observations in a two-way design

	Levels	F_1	F_2	$\ldots$	F_j	$\ldots$	F_c	Row total	Row mean
			Factor 1 (often treatments)						
	f_1	x_{11}	x_{12}	$\ldots$	x_{1j}	$\ldots$	x_{1c}	R_1	$\bar{R}_1$
	f_2	x_{21}	x_{22}	$\ldots$	$.$	$\ldots$	x_{2c}	R_2	$\bar{R}_2$
	$.$	$.$	$.$		$.$		$.$	$.$	$.$
Factor 2	$.$	$.$	$.$		$.$		$.$	$.$	$.$
(often blocks)	$.$	$.$	$.$		$.$		$.$	$.$	$.$
	f_i	x_{i1}	x_{i2}	$\ldots$	x_{ij}	$\ldots$	x_{ic}	R_i	$\bar{R}_i$
	$.$	$.$	$.$		$.$		$.$	$.$	
	$.$	$.$	$.$		$.$		$.$	$.$	
	f_r	x_{r1}	x_{r2}	$\ldots$	x_{rj}	$\ldots$	x_{rc}	R_r	$\bar{R}_r$
Column total		C_1	C_2	$\ldots$	C_j	$\ldots$	C_c	T	
Column mean		$\bar{C}_1$	$\bar{C}_2$	$\ldots$	$\bar{C}_j$	$\ldots$	$\bar{C}_c$		$\bar{x} = T/(r.c)$

where $R_i = \sum\limits_{j=1}^{c} x_{ij}$ and $\bar{R}_i = R_i/c$

$C_j = \sum\limits_{i=1}^{r} x_{ij}$ and $\bar{C}_j = C_j/r$

and $\quad T = \sum\limits_{i=1}^{r} R_i = \sum\limits_{j=1}^{c} C_j.$

Additivity

It is assumed that the row and column effects are constant and *additive*. This implies that apart from experimental errors, the difference in effect between any two rows is the same for all columns, and vice versa. The assumption of additivity is made because of its simplicity and because it is often a good approximation to more complex types of relationship.

Remark: If the row and column effects are not additive, then an *interaction* is present between these effects and it must be investigated. The interaction in a two-way table is a measure of the extent to which the effect on the variable of interest of changing the level of one factor depends on the level(s) of the other. A study of interactions is only feasible when there is replication in the cells of Table 9.2. The reader is referred to Armitage, P. (1987), pp. 257–263, for a full discussion.

Estimates of the population variance, σ^2

1. Within groups. It is *assumed* that the observations are normally distributed with constant variance, σ^2. This implies that the error terms, or residuals, are *normally distributed* with the same *constant variance, σ^2*. In order to evaluate the residual for each cell of Table 9.2, it is necessary to remove the relevant row and column effects from each reading. The row effect for the reading x_{ij} is removed by subtracting the relevant row mean, $\bar{R}_i$, from it. If this procedure is repeated for all the readings, the resulting table contains column effects and error but no row effects. If the column means of this second table are then calculated (i.e. these are $\sum\limits_{i=1}^{r} (x_{ij}-\bar{R}_i)/r = \bar{C}_j-\bar{x}$ for $j = 1, 2, \ldots, c$) and each is subtracted from the entries in the corresponding column of the second table, a third table is produced which contains only error. The entry in the ijth cell of this final table is thus of the form

$$(x_{ij}-\bar{R}_i)-(\bar{C}_j-\bar{x}) = x_{ij}-\bar{R}_i-\bar{C}_j+\bar{x}.$$

These entries are called *residuals*. Their true mean is zero and they add to zero along each row and down each column, apart from rounding errors.

If $\sum\limits_{i}^{r}\sum\limits_{j}^{c}$ denotes the sum of all terms, then the error variance, σ^2, is estimated by

$$s^2 = \sum\limits_{i}^{r}\sum\limits_{j}^{c}(x_{ij}-\bar{R}_i-\bar{C}_j+\bar{x})^2/[(r-1)(c-1)]$$

with $(r-1)(c-1)$ degrees of freedom [when there are $(r-1)(c-1)$ entries in the two-way table of residuals (excluding all those in the last row and column), the omitted entries are determined by the fact that all the marginal totals are zero. Thus the number of unrestricted or independent quantities, and hence the degrees of freedom of s^2, are $(r-1)(c-1)$]. s^2 is often called the *residual mean square*.

2. Betweeen groups. The derivation of an alternative expression for the estimate of σ^2, under the null hypothesis that the column means (or equivalently, the row means) are equal, is analogous to that shown in the one-way analysis of variance (see pp. 96–98). Thus, under the appropriate null hypothesis, σ^2 can be estimated by

$$s_C^2 = r \sum_{j=1}^{c} (\bar{C}_j - \bar{x})^2/(c-1) \text{ with } c-1 \text{ degrees of freedom}$$

or

$$s_R^2 = c \sum_{i=1}^{r} (\bar{R}_i - \bar{x})^2/(r-1) \text{ with } r-1 \text{ degrees of freedom.}$$

s_C^2 and s_R^2 are often called the *between column* and *between row mean squares,* respectively.

Ratio of estimated variances

The two null hypotheses of equality of the c column means and of the r row means are tested by determining the relevant ratios s_C^2/s^2 and s_R^2/s^2, analogous to the procedure in the one-way analysis of variance (see pp. 97–98).

Tests of hypotheses

(Equality of c population means of factor 1 (μ_1, μ_2, . . . , μ_c) and of r population means of factor 2 (γ_1, γ_2, . . . , γ_r) in a two-way analysis of variance)

1. Specify H_0^C: $\mu_1 = \mu_2 = \ldots = \mu_c = \mu$, say. If both factors are of intrinsic interest, also specify H_0^R: $\gamma_1 = \gamma_2 = \ldots = \gamma_r = \gamma$, say.
2. Specify the alternative hypotheses.
H_1^C: the μ_j are not all equal ($j = 1, 2, \ldots, c$)
H_1^R: the γ_i are not all equal ($i = 1, 2, \ldots, r$).
3. Collect the sample data appropriately. In a randomised block design in which one factor (say factor 1, representing the c treatments) is of paramount interest, randomly allocate the experimental units within each of the r blocks to the c treatments. However, if each block comprises one individual, then the order in which that subject receives each treatment is determined randomly (see within-patient studies, p. 97).

4. Present the data in a table of the form of Table 9.2. It may be possible to plot the data, depending on its nature and quantity. For example, for a randomised block design, Fig. 8.3 (relevant to the paired *t*-test) could be modified to include more than two groups (i.e. levels of factor 1).

An alternative approach to investigating the data is a study of the *residuals* (see p. 103 for their derivation). These residuals should not exhibit any striking patterns, and, if they do, this may indicate the presence of an interaction.

5. Consider the test statistic for H_0^C

$$T_{10} = s_C^2/s^2,$$

where

$$s_C^2 = r \sum_{j=1}^{c} (\bar{C}_j - \bar{x})^2/(c-1)$$

and

$$s^2 = \sum_{i=1}^{r} \sum_{j=1}^{c} (x_{ij} - \bar{R}_i - \bar{C}_j + \bar{x})^2/[(r-1)(c-1)].$$

This test statistic has an *F*-distribution with $\nu_1 = c-1$ and $\nu_2 = (r-1)(c-1)$ degrees of freedom.

Similarly, consider the test statistic for H_0^R

$$T_{11} = s_R^2/s^2$$

where

$$s_R^2 = c \sum_{i=1}^{r} (\bar{R}_i - \bar{x})^2/(r-1).$$

This test statistic has an *F*-distribution with $\nu_1 = r-1$ and $\nu_2 = (r-1)(c-1)$ degrees of freedom.

6. Compute the values, T_{10C} and (if required) T_{11C}, of these test statistics. They can be computed quite easily using only a calculator. In particular,

    a. s_C^2 is obtained by applying the usual variance formula to the column means $\bar{C}_j (j = 1, 2, \ldots, c)$ and then multiplying by r. An analogous procedure is performed for s_R^2.

Furthermore,

$$(c-1)s_C^2 = \sum^c C_j^2/r - T^2/N$$

and

$$(r-1)s_R^2 = \sum^r R_i^2/c - T^2/N.$$

b. It can be shown that

$$(r-1)(c-1)s^2 = \sum_i^r \sum_j^c (x_{ij} - \bar{x})^2 - (r-1)s_R^2 - (c-1)s_C^2$$

$$= \sum_i^r \sum_j^c x_{ij}^2 - T^2/N - (r-1)s_R^2 - (c-1)s_C^2$$

where $= \sum_i^r \sum_j^c$ denotes the sum of all terms.

7. Determine the critical regions from tables of the F-distribution (Table A4). For a one-tailed test at the $100\alpha\%$ level of significance, reject H_0^C if $T_{10C} > F_{c-1, (r-1)(c-1)}(\alpha)$, $P < \alpha$ and reject H_0^R if $T_{11C} > F_{r-1, (r-1)(c-1)}(\alpha)$, $P < \alpha$. Do not reject H_0^C and H_0^R otherwise.

Two-way analysis of variance for two groups

When there are only two groups (i.e. $c = 2$), the F-test is equivalent to the paired t-test (see pp. 87–89). In particular, it can be shown that $T_{10} = T_7^2$, i.e., the test statistic for the two-way analysis of variance is equal to the square of the test statistic for the paired t-test. This is an analogous relationship to that between the test statistic for the one-way analysis of variance and that for the two-sample t-test (see pp. 77–78).

More complex designs

Although no other designs are discussed in depth, an indication of the structure of some more complex designs is considered useful. The reader is referred to Cox, D. R. (1958) and Kempthorne, O. (1952) for full details.

1. Completely crossed designs

In a completely crossed design every level of each factor appears with every level of all other factors. When there are p factors it is sometimes called a *p-way classification*.

For a two-way classification, with r levels of one factor and c levels of the other, the data are typically presented in a table with r rows and c columns, and the classification is often termed an $r \times c$ *classification*. A *randomised block design* is an example of a two-way classification with one factor defining treatments and the other blocks of units.

2. Hierarchical (nested) classification

A form of design in which two (or more) factors are present and ordered hierarchically. Each level of one factor is associated with a *different* set of levels of the second factor, which is associated with a different set of levels of the third factor, etc. A diagrammatic representation of a two-factor hierarchical design is shown in Fig. 9.2. Each of the levels of the main factor has a *separate* subgrouping of the levels of the subgroup factor. This contrasts with the *common* row grouping of every column category in a two-way cross classification.

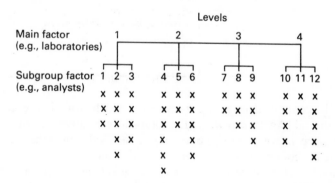

Fig. 9.2 Diagrammatic representation of a two-factor hierarchical design (each cross represents an observation).

3. Latin square

An experimental design in which the differences between n (say) levels can be tested separately for each of three factors.

The latin square may be viewed as an extension of the randomised block design. The treatments in a randomised block design are grouped into blocks so as to reduce errors in the treatment comparisons. The treatments in a latin square design are grouped into replicates in two different ways so as to allow simultaneously for two extraneous sources of variation, and hence increase the precision of the treatment comparisons.

The latin-square design is balanced with the levels of two of the factors (usually representing major sources of variation) depicted by the rows and columns of an $n \times n$ table. The levels of the third factor (usually representing treatments) are arranged such that each level of this factor appears once in each row and once in each column of the table.

A typical latin square with four levels of each factor is shown in Table 9.3, where A, B, C and D are the four levels of the third factor.

Table 9.3 Typical 4×4 latin square design for four treatments, A, B, C and D

		Factor 1			
		1	2	3	4
	1	A	B	C	D
Factor 2	2	B	A	D	C
	3	C	D	A	B
	4	D	C	B	A

In general, if there are n levels of each factor, then each cell of the table with n rows and n columns represents one of the n^2 different factor level combinations to be used. Since there are n^3 possible combinations (i.e. three factors, each at n levels), the latin square design represents a considerable saving over a three-way design. The price paid for the reduction (to $1/n$th) of experimental effort is ignorance of interactions. However, sometimes latin squares are replicated so as to increase the precision of the estimates and to enable interactions to be studied.

4. Incomplete randomised block

A randomised block is incomplete if it contains less than a complete replication of treatments, i.e. the number of units in each block is less than the number of treatments. The reduction of block size is sometimes necessary because of practical limitations and is advantageous because it increases flexibility and may well reduce residual variation. Furthermore, such a design is *balanced* (i.e. it is a balanced incomplete block, BIB) if each block contains the same number of units, each treatment occurs the same number of times in all and if each pair of treatments occurs together in the same number of blocks. See Table 9.4.

Table 9.4 Example of a BIB design for four treatments in blocks of three plots (each cross represents an observation)

Treatments	Blocks			
	I	II	III	IV
A	×	×	×	
B	×	×		×
C	×		×	×
D		×	×	×

5. Factorial experiments

A factorial design is one in which all, or nearly all, the combinations of the different levels of a set of factors are of interest (*note*: the particular combination of one level from each factor is called a 'treatment'). By analogy, all the factors are of intrinsic interest rather than one or more representing some form of blocking. In the factorial design, the main effect of each factor [i.e. the effects of the different levels of that factor averaged over the levels of the other factor(s)] and the various two-factor, three-factor (etc. as applicable) interactions can be investigated simultaneously.

An *example* of a factorial experiment with three factors each at two levels is shown in Table 9.5. *Note*: a completely crossed design has the structure of a simple factorial experiment. For example, a cross classification with two factors, one at r levels and the other at c levels is an $r \times c$ factorial design. If $r = c$, then this design is called an r^2 factorial design.

Instead of designing a factorial experiment to evaluate the effect

Table 9.5 Example of a $2\times2\times2 = 2^3$ factorial experiment with factors A, B, C each at two levels (suffices 0 and 1). Each cross represents an observation

	A_0		A_1	
	B_0	B_1	B_0	B_1
C_0	×	×	×	×
C_1	×	×	×	×

Notes:
(1) The observations are usually obtained in random order within the limitations of the experimental procedure.
(2) For example:
A_0/A_1 = standard/test preparation.
B_0/B_1 = low/high dose.
C_0/C_1 = time of administration (a.m./p.m.).

of various factors on the characteristic of interest, an *alternative* approach is to estimate the effect of each factor whilst keeping the levels of the other factors constant (at arbitrary chosen levels defining one factor combination of the remaining factors), i.e. by devoting a separate experiment, with restricted opportunity for generalisation, to each factor.

Factorial experiments have the *advantages* of:

a. Generally needing fewer observations than the non-factorial experiment to obtain the same precision to estimate the factor effects.

b. Enabling interactions between the factors to be investigated.

c. Allowing the range of validity of the conclusions to be extended by the insertion of additional factors.

However, factorial experiments are often complex and difficult to organise. They are not used that often in clinical medicine because it is usually difficult to find enough suitable patients to compare more than two or three factor combinations.

There are various *devices* which can be adopted in factorial experiments to improve their efficiency and/or meet practical requirements, e.g. to increase accuracy, to reduce cost and time of experimentation, etc. These devices include confounding and the use of split plots.

Examples

One-way analysis of variance

It is of interest to determine whether the presence of an intra-ventricular pressure gradient impairs left ventricular emptying in patients with hypertrophic cardiomyopathy. A study was performed by Siegel, R. J. and Criley, J. M. (1985) which categorised the patients into three groups; those with no gradient (Group 1), those with an inducible gradient (Group 2) and those with a resting gradient (Group 3). Let μ_i be the mean left ventricular ejection fraction (%) in the ith group ($i = 1, 2, 3$).

1. H_0: $\mu_1 = \mu_2 = \mu_3 = \mu$, say.
2. H_1: the μ_i are not all equal.
3. A random sample of individuals is selected from each of three groups. The data are presented in Table E8.3.
4. It was considered appropriate to start by investigating the underlying assumptions of the one-way analysis of variance, namely those of normality and homoscedasticity (constant variance).

The data are plotted in Fig. E8.3, from which it can be seen that the observations in each group are skewed to the left and are, therefore, not normally distributed. However, since the F-test in the one-way analysis of variance is a robust test, insensitive to non-normality of the data, the use of this test is still considered satisfactory.

Because of the non-normality of the data, it is inappropriate to compare the group variances formally by the methods discussed in Chapter 8, pp. 81–82. However, by inspecting Fig. E8.3, and noting that the range of observations within each group does not appear to differ in the three groups, there is an indication that assumption of homoscedasticity is not unreasonable.

5. Consider

$$T_9 = s_b^2/s_w^2$$

where

$$(k-1)s_b^2 = \sum_{i=1}^{k} T_i^2/n_i - T^2$$

$$= [(604^2/8) + (851^2/10) + (1382^2/15)] - 2837^2/33$$

$$= 1454.336$$

so

$$s_b^2 = 1454.336/(3-1) = 727.168$$

and

$$s_w^2 = \sum_{i=1}^{k} (n_i-1)s_i^2/(N-k)$$

$$= [7(62.286)+9(80.76^{\cdot})+14(41.124)]/(33-3)$$

$$= 57.953$$

6. $\qquad T_{9C} = 1454.336/57.953 = 12.58.$

7. From the table of the F-distribution (Table A4), $F_{2,30}(0.001)$ = 8.77. Hence $T_{9C} > F_{2,30}(0.001)$ since $12.58 > 8.77$. Thus reject H_0 that there is no difference between the mean left ventricular ejection fractions in the three groups ($P < 0.001$) (*note*: the differences between specific means are investigated in the Examples to Chapter 8, p. 89).

Two-way analysis of variance

A randomised block experiment was designed to show whether the response (weal size) to intradermal injection of antibody followed by antigen depends on the method of preparation of the antibody. Four different preparations (A, B, C and D) were tested.

Table E9.1 Weal diameters (x_{ij}; $i,j = 1, 2, 3, 4$) using four antibody preparations in guinea pigs

Guinea pig (i)	Antibody preparation (j)				Total	Mean ($\bar{R}_i$)
	A($j = 1$)	B($j = 2$)	C($j = 3$)	D($j = 4$)		
1	41	61	62	43	207	51.75
2	48	68	62	48	226	56.50
3	53	70	66	53	242	60.50
4	56	72	70	52	250	62.50
Total	198	271	260	196	925	
Mean ($\bar{C}_j$)	49.5	67.75	65.0	49.0		

Source: Čoloquhoun, D. (1971) *Lectures on Biostatistics* Oxford: Oxford University Press; p. 199.

Each preparation was injected once into each of four randomly selected quinea pigs. Let μ_i be the mean weal size for the ith preparation ($i = 1, 2, 3, 4$).

1. H_0^C: $\mu_1 = \mu_2 = \mu_3 = \mu_4 = \mu$, say.
2. H_1^C: the μ_i are not all equal.
· 3. The preparation to be given to each of the four sites on each animal was decided at random.
4. The results are presented in Table E9.1. Table E9.2 contains preparation effects and error but no animal effects, and is obtained by subtracting the relevant preparation means from the readings in Table E9.1. Finally, Table E9.3 is a table of residuals. It contains only error and is obtained by subtracting the relevant column means in Table E9.2 from the entries in Table E9.2. No particular pattern

Table E9.2 Table E9.1 with relevant row means of Table E9.1 subtracted from each reading ($x_{ij} - \bar{R}_i$; $i, j = 1, 2, 3, 4$)

| Guinea pig (i) | Antibody preparation (j) | | | | |
	A	B	C	D	Total
1	−10.75	9.25	10.25	−8.75	0.00
2	−8.50	11.50	5.50	−8.50	0.00
3	−7.50	9.50	5.50	−7.50	0.00
4	−6.50	9.50	7.50	−10.50	0.00
Total	−33.25	39.75	28.75	−35.25	0.00
Mean	−8.3125	9.9375	7.1875	−8.8125	

Table E9.3 Table E9.2 with relevant column means of Table E9.2 subtracted from each entry ($x_{ij} - \bar{R}_i - \bar{C}_j + \bar{x}$; $i, j = 1, 2, 3, 4$)

| Guinea pig (i) | Antibody preparation (j) | | | | |
	A	B	C	D	Total
1	−2.4375	−0.6875	3.0625	0.0625	0.0000
2	−0.1875	1.5625	−1.6875	0.3125	0.0000
3	0.8125	−0.4375	−1.6875	1.3125	0.0000
4	1.8125	−0.4375	−0.3125	−1.6875	0.0000
Total	0.0000	0.0000	0.0000	0.0000	0.0000

emerges from this table of residuals containing nine negative values and seven positive values.

5. Consider $T_{10} = s_C^2/s^2$

where $\qquad s_C^2 = 4 \sum_{j=1}^{4} (\bar{C}_j - \bar{x})^2/(4-1)$

$$= 4(99.0573)$$

$$= 396.2292,$$

and since $(x_{ij} - \bar{R}_i - \bar{C}_j + \bar{x})$ is the ijth term in Table E9.3 of residuals,

$$s^2 = \sum_{i}^{4} \sum_{j}^{4} (\bar{x}_{ij} - \bar{R}_i - \bar{C}_j + \bar{x})^2/[(4-1)(4-1)]$$

$$= (313.0625)/9$$

$$= 3.6736.$$

6. $\qquad T_{10C} = (396.2292)/(3.6736) = 107.85.$

7. From the table of the F-distribution (Table A4) $F_{3,9}(0.001) = 13.90$. Hence $T_{10C} > F_{3,9}(0.001)$ since $107.85 > 13.90$. Thus reject H_0^C that there is no difference in the mean weal diameters in the four antibody preparations ($P < 0.001$).

Note: Coloquhoun shows (using Scheffés method) that preparations B and C both give larger responses than preparations A and D ($P < 0.001$), but that no difference can be detected between A and D ($P > 0.05$), or between B and C ($P > 0.05$).

Chapter 10
The Chi-square Test

Introduction

The chi-square (χ^2) test relates to the *frequencies* of occurrence of individuals in the categories of one or more variables. The actual qualitative or quantitative values of the variable(s) are not relevant to the test, except in defining the categories of interest and in allocating the individuals to those categories.

Application

In its basic form, the χ^2 test determines whether the observed frequencies of individuals with given characteristics differ significantly from the frequencies which would be expected under some theory or hypothesis. The two important applications are goodness of fit and analysis of contingency tables.

Goodness of fit

An observed frequency distribution is compared to a theoretical distribution (e.g. binomial, normal). The test evaluates how well the observed frequencies in different categories agree with those expected if the data possessed the prescribed theoretical distribution. The details are not discussed here for the procedure is arduous so that it (or alternatives to it) is generally performed using computer packages, and in any case, it is often unwarranted. In particular, the assumption of normality of data prescribed in many tests of hypotheses can be approximately validated by simple plots and inspection by eye.

Analysis of contingency tables

Only two-way contingency tables are considered. A two-way contingency table is a table in which the rows represent the r (say) mutually exclusive categories of one variable and the columns

Chapter 10

represent the *c* (say) mutually exclusive categories of another variable. The cell corresponding to a particular row category and column category contains the number of individuals in both of these categories. The contingency table is thus a table of *frequencies* showing how the total frequency is distributed among the cells of the table. The table is usually constructed for the purpose of studying the relation between the two variables of classification. The χ^2 test is a means of testing the hypothesis that the two variables are *independent*, i.e. no relationship exists between them.

Definition of the χ^2 statistic

Consider *k* mutually exclusive events (e.g. an event is a single category in a goodness-of-fit test and an event is a pair of categories, one from each of two variables, in a test of association in a contingency table). Suppose that in a sample of *n* observations, the observed frequency of occurrence of the *i*th event ($i = 1, 2, \ldots, k$) is O_i and that its expected frequency of occurrence (determined under some theory or hypothesis) is E_i. Clearly $\sum^k O_i = n$. A measure of the discrepancy existing between the observed and expected frequencies is supplied by the statistic X^2 given by

$$
\begin{aligned}
X^2 &= \frac{(O_1 - E_1)^2}{E_1} + \frac{(O_2 - E_2)^2}{E_2} + \ldots + \frac{(O_k - E_k)^2}{E_k} \\
&= \sum_{i=1}^{k} \frac{(O_i - E_i)^2}{E_i} \\
&= \sum^k \frac{O_i^2}{E_i} - n \quad \text{(for ease of calculation)}.
\end{aligned}
$$

The squaring of the differences overcomes the nullifying effect of the opposing signs, and dividing by the expected frequencies standardises the magnitude.

Implications

1. If $X^2 = 0$ (highly unlikely)
The observed and expected frequencies agree exactly and there is no evidence against the hypothesis under which the expected frequencies are calculated.

2. If $X^2 > 0$

If X^2 is small, the implication is that the observed and expected frequencies do not differ markedly, and there is no strong evidence against the hypothesis. The larger the value of X^2, the greater the discrepancy between observed and expected frequencies and the less likely it is that the hypothesis is true. There exists a *critical value* of X^2 such that any value of X^2 greater than this critical value implies disagreement between observed and expected frequencies. Since the sampling distribution of X^2 is approximated by the χ^2 *distribution* (provided the expected frequencies are not too small), the critical value is the appropriate percentage point of the χ^2 distribution. The degrees of freedom of the distribution depend on the problem under consideration.

Hypothesis test: independence of two variables in an $r \times c$ contingency table

The variables of interest are x, which is classified into c mutually exclusive categories $x_1, x_2, \ldots, x_c$ (e.g. $x =$ age, $x_1 = {} < 20$ years, $x_2 = 20$–40 years, $x_3 = {} > 40$ years), and y, which is classified into r mutually exclusive categories $y_1, y_2, \ldots, y_r$ (e.g. $y =$ blood group, $y_1 = $ A, $y_2 = $ B, $y_3 = $ AB, $y_4 = $ O). The general procedure for testing an hypothesis (see Chapter 7) is followed.

1. Define H_0: the classifications of x and y are independent.
2. Define H_1: the classifications of x and y are not independent. There is an association between the levels (categories) of x and y; high levels of x are associated with high levels of y (positive association) or high levels of x are association with low levels of y (negative association).
3. Collect a random sample of n individuals from the population. Determine for every category of x, the number of individuals belonging to each category of y.
4. Instead of plotting the data, collect the frequencies into a contingency table of the form shown in Table 10.1.
5. Consider the test statistic

$$X^2 = \sum_i^r \sum_j^c (O_{ij} - E_{ij})^2 / E_{ij}$$

where $E_{ij} = (R_i C_j)/n$. In *words*, if the expected frequency of a particular cell is defined as the product of the marginal frequencies

Chapter 10

Table 10.1 General form of $r \times c$ contingency table displaying observed frequencies

		Variable x						Row marginal total
		x_1	x_2	. . .	x_j	. . .	x_c	
	y_1				.			R_1
	y_2				.			R_2
	.				.			.
Variable y	y_i	. . . . .			O_{ij}	. . . . .		R_i
	.				.			.
	y_r				.			R_r
Column marginal total		C_1 C_2 . . .			C_j		. . . C_c	n

O_{ij} is the cell frequency for ith row and jth column.

$R_i = \sum_j O_{ij}$ is the row marginal frequency for ith row.

$C_j = \sum_i O_{ij}$ is the column marginal frequency for jth column.

$n = \sum_i \sum_j O_{ij}$ is the total frequency.

common to the cell divided by the total frequency, then the test statistic is determined by considering for each cell, the square of the difference between the observed and the expected frequencies, divided by the expected frequency, and then summing this ratio over all cells. The sampling distribution of this statistic is approximately χ^2 on $(r-1)(c-1)$ degrees of freedom. *Note:*

a. EXPECTED FREQUENCIES
$E_{ij} = (R_i C_j)/n$ is the number of individuals that would be expected in the (i, j)th cell if H_0 were true. For if the classifications of the two variables are independent, the proportion of individuals in category y_i is the same for all categories of x. The proportion of individuals in category y_i is R_i/n and the total number of individuals in category x_j is C_j, so that under H_0, the expected number of individuals in both y_i and x_j is $C_j(R_i/n)$.

b. YATES' CORRECTION
Since the sampling distribution of X^2 is *discrete* and it is approxi-

mated by the *continuous* χ^2 distribution, a continuity correction may be applied to the test statistic to allow for the discrepancy. The effect of the continuity correction is to replace the difference between the observed and expected frequencies for each cell in the numerator of the test statistic by its absolute difference minus 1/2. The test statistic corrected for continuity is

$$X_y^2 = \sum_i^r \sum_j^c (|O_{ij}-E_{ij}|-1/2)^2/E_{ij}.$$

The continuity correction is called *Yates' correction*. It should be applied only when $r = c = 2$.

c. SMALL EXPECTED FREQUENCIES

If any of the expected frequencies are small (less than 5, say), then the sampling distribution of X^2 is not approximated by the χ^2 distribution. A new reduced contingency table should be constructed by combining any two or more adjacent rows and/or any two or more adjacent columns (the rows and/or columns being chosen so that their juncture may be meaningfully interpreted), such that the expected frequency of each cell of this new table is at least 5. The test statistic, X^2 (or X_Y^2), is then considered for this new table. An *exception* is the 2×2 table ($r = c = 2$) which can be reduced no further. *Fisher's exact test*, which makes no distributional approximations, is then warranted. The reader is referred to Armitage, P. (1987), pp. 91–132, for a discussion of the test.

6. Compute the value, X_C^2 (or X_{YC}^2), of the test statistic from the sample data.

7. Determine the critical region from tables of the χ^2 distribution (Table A2). For a test at the $100\alpha\%$ level of significance, reject H_0 if X_C^2 (or X_{YC}^2) $> \chi^2_{(r-1)(c-1)}(\alpha)$, $P < \alpha$. Do not reject H_0 otherwise, $P > \alpha$.

The fourfold (2×2) table

Simple formulae for computing X^2 and X_Y^2

A special case of the $r\times c$ contingency table is the fourfold table in which $r = c = 2$. As this occurs frequently in practice, simple formulae for calculating X^2 and X_Y^2 are given. The notation used is explained in Table 10.2.

Provided that the expected frequencies in all cells are large enough, the sampling distribution of X^2 (or X_Y^2) is approximately χ^2 on one degree of freedom.

Table 10.2 Observed frequencies in a fourfold table

		Variable x		
		x_1	x_2	Row marginal total
Variable y	y_1	a	b	$R_1 = a+b$
	y_2	c	d	$R_2 = c+d$
Column marginal total		$C_1 = a+c$	$C_2 = b+d$	$n = a+b+c+d$

$$X^2 = \frac{n(ad-bc)^2}{R_1 R_2 C_1 C_2} = \left(\frac{a}{R_1} - \frac{c}{R_2}\right)\left(\frac{a}{C_1} - \frac{b}{C_2}\right)n$$

$$X_Y^2 = \frac{n(|ad-bc|-n/2)^2}{R_1 R_2 C_1 C_2}.$$

Hypothesis test: equality of two proportions (π_1, π_2)

Independent samples

The χ^2 test of independence of the two variables in a fourfold table provides a test for the equality of two proportions when these proportions are estimated from two independent samples. Suppose that the two independent samples are distinguished by the classifications of the x variable and that interest is centred on the equality of the proportions of y_1-individuals in the two samples. If the classifications of the two variables, x and y, are independent, then the proportion of individuals in category y_1 out of the total number of individuals in both y categories is the same in category x_1 [the proportion π_1, estimated in the sample by $p_1 = a/(a+c)$] and in category x_2 [the proportion π_2 estimated in the sample by $p_2 = b/(b+d)$]. Thus an alternative expression of the null hypothesis of independence of the classifications of the two variables is $H_0: \pi_1 = \pi_2$.

Paired samples (McNemar's test)

Frequencies should not be presented in a fourfold table when the two samples (identified by the classifications of the x variable, say) consist of paired individuals. Instead, some indication should be given, for all pairs, of the classifications of the variable of interest (y) for both members of the pair, in order that the appropriate comparison of the two relevant proportions be made. Thus if the variable of interest can be classified as either y_1 or y_2, then clearly there are four possible types of pair. These types and their frequencies of occurrence are shown in Table 10.3 and also in the two-way Table 10.4.

Table 10.3 Types of pair and their observed frequencies of occurrence in paired samples

Type	Sample 1	Sample 2	No. of pairs
1	y_1	y_1	f_1
2	y_1	y_2	f_2
3	y_2	y_1	f_3
4	y_2	y_2	f_4
Total			N

Table 10.4 Two-way table of observed frequencies of pairs of individuals

		Sample 2 y_1	Sample 2 y_2	Total pairs
Sample 1	y_1	f_1	f_2	f_1+f_2
	y_2	f_3	f_4	f_3+f_4
Total		f_1+f_3	f_2+f_4	$N = f_1+f_2+f_3+f_4$

Interest is centred on the equality of the proportions of y_1-individuals in two populations, π_1 [estimated by $(f_1+f_2)/N$ in sample 1] and π_2 [estimated by $(f_1+f_3)/N$ in sample 2]. The procedure for testing this equality is as follows:

1. Define H_0: $\pi_1 = \pi_2$.
2. Define H_1: $\pi_1 \neq \pi_2$, say.
3. Select two random samples of individuals such that each individual in one sample is matched with an individual in the other

sample. Determine, for all pairs, the classifications of the y variable for both members of a matched pair so that each pair can be typed (as in Table 10.3).

4. Instead of plotting the data, collect the frequencies of the four types of pair in a two-way table of the form shown in Table 10.4.

5. Consider the test statistic (which is corrected for continuity)

$$T_3^2 = \frac{(|f_2-f_3|-1)^2}{f_2+f_3}.$$

The sampling distribution of this test statistic for large enough (f_2+f_3) is approximately χ^2 on one degree of freedom.

Justification of the choice of T_3^2:

a. The tied type 1 (y_1y_1) and the type 4 (y_2y_2) pairs can be ignored in the test of significance since they give no relevant additional information.

b. If H_0 is true, then the population of untied pairs contains as many type 2 (y_1y_2) as type 3 (y_2y_1) pairs. Suppose the proportion of type 2 (y_1y_2) pairs in the population of untied pairs is π, estimated in the sample by $p = f_2/(f_2+f_3)$. Then under H_0, $\pi = 1/2(= \pi_0)$, and the test is of a single proportion (Chapter 7). The test statistic, corrected for continuity, is thus

$$T_3 = [|p-\pi_0|-1/(2n)]/\sqrt{\pi_0(1-\pi_0)/n},$$

where in this context, $n = f_2+f_3$. T_3 has approximately a standard normal distribution for large enough n. On substitution,

$$\begin{aligned}T_3 &= \{|f_2/(f_2+f_3)-1/2|-1/[2(f_2+f_3)]\}/\sqrt{(1/2)^2/(f_2+f_3)} \\ &= (|f_2-f_3|-1)/\sqrt{f_2+f_3}\end{aligned}$$

(i.e. this is the *sign test*; see also the Examples to Chapter 12).

c. The sampling distribution of the square of a standard normal deviate is χ^2 on one degree of freedom (see Chapter 5, p. 43). Thus the distribution of T_3^2 for large enough (f_1+f_2) is approximately χ^2 on one degree of freedom. Therefore, instead of evaluating T_3 and referring to tables of the standard normal distribution, an alternative approach to testing H_0 is to evaluate T_3^2 and refer to tables of the χ^2 distribution. This latter procedure achieves consistency of method when testing the equality of two proportions through its dependence on tables of the χ^2

distribution. (*Note:* The sampling distribution of the test statistic, X^2, whose square root is considered when testing H_0: $\pi_1 = \pi_2$ using two independent samples, is approximately χ_1^2.)

6. Compute the value, T_{3C}^2, of the test statistic from the sample data.

7. Determine the critical region from tables of the χ^2 distribution (Table A2). For a test at the $100\alpha\%$ level of significance, reject H_0 if $T_{3C}^2 > \chi_1^2(\alpha)$, $P < \alpha$. Do not reject H_0 otherwise, $P > \alpha$. *Note:* The difference in the proportions of y_1-individuals is estimated in the samples by

$$[(f_1+f_2)/N-(f_1+f_3)/N] = (f_2-f_3)/N$$

with a standard error estimated by $\sqrt{(f_2+f_3)}/N$. Thus the 95% *confidence interval* for the difference in the two proportions, using the usual normal theory, is

$$[(f_2-f_3)/N-1.96\sqrt{(f_2+f_3)}/N, (f_2-f_3)/N+1.96\sqrt{(f_2+f_3)}/N].$$

Hypothesis test: equality of more than two proportions ($\pi_1, \pi_2 \ldots \pi_k$)

When more than two like parameters (e.g., means, proportions or variances) are to be compared it is tempting to perform multiple tests on all pairwise comparisons (e.g. on all combinations of two proportions). This procedure should be avoided (see discussion on pp. 78–79) as the more tests that are performed the greater the probability of finding a significant difference (in the absence of a real difference) purely by chance.

When the equality of more than two *means* is in question, one solution is to perform an analysis of variance and follow this by pairwise comparisons of logical interest only if the former analysis is significant. When attention centres on the equality of more than two *proportions* in *independent* samples, the overall significance test discussed below provides an initial solution to the problem. If this test is significant, it should be followed by pairwise comparisons of proportions of *a priori* interest or, perhaps, by a linear trend analysis.

Suppose the k independent samples are distinguished by the classifications of the x variable, and that the investigation is concerned with testing the equality of the proportions of y_1-individuals in the k populations, when the y variable is categorised as either y_1 or y_2. Let π_i be the proportion of y_1-individuals in the population classified as x_i ($i = 1, 2, \ldots, k$). The procedure for testing the equality of the k proportions is as follows:

1. Define H_0: $\pi_1 = \pi_2 = \ldots = \pi_k = \pi$, say.
2. Define H_1: Not all the π_i ($i = 1, 2, \ldots, k$) are equal.
3. Select k random samples of individuals, one from each of the k populations. Determine for each sample, the classifications of the y variable; i.e. the *number* of individuals classified as y_1 and as y_2.
4. Instead of plotting the data, collect the frequencies in a two-way table of the form shown in Table 10.5.

Table 10.5 Observed frequencies in a two-way table

		Variable x					Row marginal total
		x_1	x_2	. . .	x_i . . .	x_k	
Variable y y_1		r_1	r_2	. . .	r_i . . .	r_k	R
y_2		$n_1 - r_1$	$n_2 - r_2$	. . .	$n_i - r_i$ . . .	$n_k - r_k$	$n - R$
Column marginal total		n_1	n_2	. . .	n_i . . .	n_k	n
Proportion of y_1-individuals		p_1	p_2	. . .	p_i . . .	p_k	$P = \dfrac{R}{n}$

Note
    a. $p_i = r_i / n_i$, $i = 1, 2, \ldots, k$.
    b. See also discussion of binomial distribution pp. 132–133 and distribution of sample proportion pp. 42–43 for properties of p_i.
    c. Table 10.5 is a $2 \times k$ contingency table (see pp. 117–119) containing k columns, rather than c, to conform with the analogous comparison of k means in the one-way analysis of variance (see p. 96).
5. The χ^2 test of independence of the classifications of the two variables x and y in a $2 \times k$ contingency table (see pp. 117–119 for details of the test for the more generalised $r \times c$ contingency table; in this instance, take $r = 2$, $c = k$) provides a test of equality of the k proportions.

Justification: The χ^2 test of independence of two variables in a 2×2 contingency table is equivalent to a test of equality of two proportions when these proportions are estimated in two independent samples (see p. 120). This concept may be extended to the simultaneous comparison of several proportions.

Note: It can be shown quite simply (see Armitage, P. (1987), pp. 206–207) that an *equivalent formula* for the test statistic, when $r = 2$ and $c = k$, is

$$X^2 = \sum_{i=1}^{k} \frac{(p_i - P)^2}{P(1-P)/n_i} = \frac{\sum_{i=1}^{k} r_i p_i - RP}{P(1-P)}$$

which has a χ^2 distribution with $k-1$ degrees of freedom.

Alternative justification of X^2: if the binomial estimates, p_i, are all based on the same size n, X^2 becomes $\sum_{i=1}^{k} (p_i - P)^2/[P(1-P)/n]$. The numerator is $(k-1)$ times the estimated variance of the p_i. The denominator is the estimated variance that the p_i would have if they were derived from independent samples from the same binomial distribution (i.e. under H_0). This interpretation of X^2 can be extended to the situation when the n_i vary. Then it can be seen that X^2 has approximately a χ^2 distribution with $(k-1)$ degrees of freedom (see property 4 of χ^2 distribution, p. 43) using the normal approximation to the binomial distribution and replacing the true variance of the p_i under H_0 by its estimate.

Trend in proportions

Sometimes the k classifications of the x variable fall in natural order and, as an adjunct to the procedure discussed above, it is of interest to determine whether there is a significant linear trend in the proportions of y_1-individuals from the first to the kth classification of x.

The basis of the approach is a linear regression analysis (see Chapter 11) of p_i (weighted by the sample size, n_i, on which it is based) on x_i, the value assigned to each of the categorisations of the column variable. In the absence of any *a priori* knowledge of the type of trend to be expected, these latter 'dummy' values or scores are generally chosen to be equally spaced and often centred around zero. Thus for k columns, the values $x_1 = -\frac{1}{2}(k-1)$, $x_2 = -\frac{1}{2}(k-3)$, . . . , $x_k = \frac{1}{2}(k-1)$ might be selected.

The reader is referred to Armitage, P. (1987), pp. 372–374, for a discussion of the appropriate test; and to the Examples section of this chapter for an example.

Coefficient of contingency

The χ^2 test determines only whether a relationship exists between the classifications of two variables in a contingency table. The degree of that relationship or association may be quantified by a coefficient of contingency.

$r\times c$ table

Pearson's coefficient of contingency, P
$$P = \sqrt{X^2/(X^2+n)}$$

Properties: (i) $0 \leqslant P \leqslant 1$ (considering only the positive value of the square root); (ii) $P = 0$ implies no association; (iii) the larger P, the greater the degree of association; and (iv) the upper limit of P depends on the number of categories.

Cramer's modified coefficient of contingency, C
$$C = \sqrt{X^2/[n \min(r-1, c-1)]}$$
where

$$\min (r-1, c-1) = \begin{cases} r-1 & \text{if } r \leqslant c \\ c-1 & \text{if } r \geqslant c \end{cases}$$

Properties: (i) $0 \leqslant C \leqslant 1$ (considering only the positive value of the square root); (ii) $C = 0$ implies no association; (iii) the larger C, the greater the degree of association; and (iv) $C = 1$ implies complete association.

2×2 table

The coefficient of contingency most commonly utilised is (using the notation of Table 10.2)

$$V = \frac{ad-bc}{\sqrt{(R_1R_2C_1C_2)}}.$$

Properties: (i) $-1 \leq V \leq +1$; (ii) the larger $|V|$, the greater the degree of association; (iii) $V = +1$ implies complete positive association; (iv) $V = -1$ implies complete negative association; and (v) $|V| = C$ when $r = c = 2$.

Examples

Independence of two variables in a 2×4 contingency table

It is of interest to investigate the possible association between detectable measles haemagglutination inhibitory titre and age at vaccination in schoolchildren.

1. H_0: The detectable antibody titre is independent of the age at vaccination in schoolchildren.

2. H_1: There is an association between detectable antibody titre and the age at vaccination.

3. A random sample of children from five schools in north-east metropolitan Detroit is selected. A serum sample is available for each child. The detectable measles haemagglutination inhibitory titre are observed in the children and the ages at which these children were vaccinated are noted.

4. The results are presented in Table E10.1.

5. The expected frequencies corresponding to each cell of Table E10.1 are given in Table E10.2 [3.43 = (19)(46)/(255),

Table E10.1 Detectable measles haemagglutination inhibitory titre according to age at vaccination (a 2×4 contingency table)

		Age (months)				
		< 9	9–11	12	≥ 13	Total
No. with titre	< 5	11	13	13	9	46
	≥ 5	8	41	53	107	209
Total		19	54	66	116	255

Source: Shasby, D. M. *et al* (1977) reprinted, by permission, from the *New England Journal of Medicine*, **296**, 585–589, 1977.

Table E10.2   Expected frequencies

		Age (months)				
		< 9	9–11	12	≥ 13	Total
No. with titre	< 5	3.43	9.74	11.91	20.93	46.01
	≥ 5	15.57	44.26	54.09	95.07	208.99
Total		19	54	66	116	255

Source: Table E10.1.

$15.57 = (19)(209)/255$, etc.]. Since one expected frequency has a value which is less than 5, it might be argued that it is not really appropriate to test H_0 by calculating the X^2 statistic and referring to tables of the χ^2 distribution. Instead, the observed contingency table is reduced by combining the first two age groups to form a new age group of babies vaccinated at less than 12 months. The observed frequencies are shown in Table E10.3 and the corresponding expected frequencies for this reduced table are shown in Table E10.4 [$13.17 = (73)(46)/(255)$, $59.83 = (73)(209)/(255)$, etc.].

Table E10.3   Observed frequencies in reduced table

		Age (months)			
		< 12	12	≥ 13	Total
No. with titre	< 5	24	13	9	46
	≤ 5	49	53	107	209
Total		73	66	116	255

Source: Table E10.1.

6. $X_C^2 = (24-13.17)^2/(13.17)+(49-59.83)^2/(59.83)$
$\qquad +(13-11.91)^2/(11.91)+(53-54.09)^2/(54.09)$
$\qquad +(9-20.93)^2/(20.93)+(107-95.07)^2/(95.07)$
$\quad = 8.906+1.960+ \ldots +1.497$
$\quad = 19.28.$

Table E10.4 Expected frequencies in reduced table

		Age (months)			
		< 12	12	≥ 13	Total
No. with titre	< 5	13.17	11.91	20.93	46.01
	≥ 5	59.83	54.09	95.07	208.99
Total		73	66	116	255

Source: Table E10.3.

7. From tables of the χ^2 distribution (Table A2), $\chi^2_2(0.001) = 13.82$ (*note:* degrees of freedom $= (3-1)(2-1) = 2$). Hence $X^2_C > \chi^2(0.001)$ since $19.28 > 13.82$. Thus reject H_0 that the detectable antibody titre is independent of the age at vaccination, $P < 0.001$.

Coefficient of contingency

Pearson's:

$$P = \sqrt{\frac{X^2}{X^2+n}} = \sqrt{\frac{19.28}{19.28+255}} = 0.27.$$

Cramer's:

$$C = \sqrt{\frac{X^2}{n \min (r-1, c-1)}} = \sqrt{\frac{19.28}{(255)(1)}} = 0.27.$$

The fourfold table

1. H_0: There is no association between systemic lupus erythematosus (SLE) and the prevalence of warts.

2. H_1: There is an association between SLE and the prevalence of warts.

3. A random sample of 56 SLE patients is selected from a hospital in a 2-year period. The 160 control patients are consecutive patients attending the dermatology outpatient department or admitted to the hospital for various cutaneous tests during the period. Patients admitted because of warts are excluded from the study. Neither the age distribution nor the sex distribution of the SLE and control groups differ significantly. The prevalence of warts in both groups is recorded.

Table E10.5 Observed frequencies (fourfold table)

	Warts	No warts	Total
SLE	25	31	56
Controls	19	141	160
Total	44	172	216

Source: Johansson, E., Pyrhönen, S., and Rostila, T. (1977). Warts and wart virus antibodies in patients with systemic lupus erythematosus. *Br. med. J.* **i**, 74–76.

Table E10.6 Expected frequencies

	Warts	No warts	Total
SLE	11.41	44.59	56.00
Controls	32.59	127.41	160.00
Total	44.00	172.00	216.00

Source: Table E10.5.

4. The results are presented in Table E10.5.

5. The expected frequencies corresponding to each cell of Table E10.5 are given in Table E10.6 [$11.41 = (44)(56)/(216)$, $31 = (172)(56)/(216)$, etc.].

6. Using Yates' correction

$$X_{YC}^2 = \sum\sum(|O_{ij}-E_{ij}|-1/2)^2/E_{ij}$$
$$= (|25-11.41|-1/2)^2/(11.41)+(|31-44.59|-1/2)^2/(44.59)$$
$$+(|19-32.59|-1/2)^2/(32.59)+(|14-127.41|-1/2)^2/(127.41)$$
$$= 25.48.$$

Alternatively:

$$X_{YC}^2 = n(|ad-bc|-n/2)^2/(R_1\,R_2\,C_1\,C_2)$$
$$= 216[|(25)(141)-(31)(19)|-(216)/2]^2/[(56)(160)(44)(172)]$$
$$= 216(2936-108)^2/(67809280)$$
$$= 25.48.$$

7. Using tables of the χ^2 distribution (Table A2), $\chi_1^2(0.001) = 10.83$ [*note:* degrees of freedom $= (2-1)(2-1) = 1$]. Hence $X_{YC}^2 > \chi_1^2(0.001)$ since $25.48 > 10.83$. Thus reject H_0 that there is no association between SLE and the prevalence of warts, $P < 0.001$.

Remark: It should be noted that this χ^2 test is investigating whether the *proportion* of SLE patients with warts is the same as the *proportion* of an independent group of control patients with warts, these proportions being estimated in the samples by $25/56 = 0.45$ and $19/160 = 0.12$, respectively.

Coefficient of contingency

$$V = \frac{ad - bc}{\sqrt{(R_1 R_2 C_1 C_2)}} = \frac{(25)(141) - (31)(19)}{\sqrt{[(56)(160)(44)(172)]}} = 0.36.$$

McNemar's test (paired samples)

1. H_0: There is no association between appendicectomy and maturity-onset diabetes, i.e. the prevalence of appendicectomy among patients with maturity-onset diabetes is the same as that among a control group without maturity-onset diabetes.

2. H_1: There is an association between appendicectomy and maturity-onset diabetes.

3. A random sample of 251 individuals (104 men and 147 women) aged 40 years and upwards, who have not been diagnosed as suffering from diabetes mellitus before the age of 40, is selected from an outpatient diabetic clinic in a hospital. A random sample of 251 controls is selected. They are individuals matched with the diabetics for sex and age, attending the accident and emergency department of the hospital, and in whom diabetes is excluded. Whether or not each patient has had an appendicectomy is determined.

4. The results are presented in Table E10.7.

Table E10.7 Appendicectomy state of diabetics and controls

	Diabetics		
Controls	Appendicectomy	No appendicectomy	Total pairs
Appendicectomy	8	48	56
No appendicectomy	34	161	195
Total	42	209	251

Source: Corridan, J., O'Regan, J. P., and O'Sullivan, D. J. (1977) Diabetes and appendicectomy: testing a hypothesis. *Br. med. J.* **i,** 1135.

5. Consider the test statistic

$$T_3^2 = (|f_2 - f_3| - 1)^2 / (f_2 + f_3).$$

6.
$$\begin{aligned}
T_{3C}^2 &= (|48 - 34| - 1)^2 / (48 + 34) \\
&= (13)^2 / (82) \\
&= 2.1.
\end{aligned}$$

7. Using tables of the χ^2 distribution (Table A2), $\chi_1^2(0.05) = 3.84$. Hence $T_{3C}^2 < \chi_1^2(0.05)$ since $2.1 < 3.84$. Thus do not reject H_0 that there is no association between appendicectomy and maturity-onset diabetes, $P > 0.05$.

Note: The difference in the two proportions is estimated by

$$(f_2 - f_3)/N = (48 - 34)/(251) = 0.056.$$

with a standard error estimated by

$$\sqrt{(f_2 + f_3)}/N = \sqrt{(48 + 34)}/(251) = 0.036.$$

The approximate 95% *confidence interval* for the difference in the two proportions is

$$[0.056 - (1.96)(0.036), \; 0.056 + (1.96)(0.036)] = [0.015, 0.127].$$

Equality of more than 2 proportions

The example on pp. 127–129, investigating the possible association between detectable measles haemagglutination inhibitory titre and age at vaccination in schoolchildren, approached the problem by testing the null hypothesis of no association between them. An alternative but equally acceptable specification of the null hypothesis is that the proportions of schoolchildren having a detectable measles haemagglutination inhibitory titre of less than 5 are equal in different age-at-vaccination categories. Using the data from Table E10.3, the estimated proportions of children with titre less than 5 in the three age-at-vaccination categories, < 12, 12 and $\geqslant 13$ months are $24/73 = 0.329$, $13/66 = 0.197$ and $9/116 = 0.078$, respectively, with an overall proportion, if the null hypothesis is true, estimated by $46/255 = 0.180$. Applying the simpler formula for the test statistic, namely $X^2 = (\sum r_i p_i - RP)/[P(P-1)]$, so that its calculated value is

$$X_C^2 = (11.1493 - 1.8039)/1.4785 = 19.28$$

produces an identical result to that obtained using the more general formula. Thus, by referring to Table A2 using 2 degrees of freedom, the null hypothesis that the proportions are equal is rejected. $P < 0.001$.

Note: It is considered expedient to perform the test for a linear trend in proportions in this example although details of the test are not described in the text in which only a reference is provided. The test statistic is

$$X_1^2 = \frac{n\left[n\sum_{i=1}^{k} r_i x_i - R\sum_{i=1}^{k} n_i x_i\right]^2}{R(n-R)\left[N\sum_{i=1}^{k} n_i x_i^2 - \left(\sum_{i=1}^{k} n_i x_i\right)^2\right]},$$

using the notation of Table 10.5. This is calculated as $255[255(-15)-46(43)]^2/\{46(209)[255(189)-43^2]\} = 19.27$ when x_1, x_2 and x_3 are -1, 0 and 1, respectively (*note:* -1, 0 and 1 are the scores assigned to x_1, x_2 and x_3 in the absence of any accurate measure of age and assuming equally spaced age intervals). The sampling distribution of this test statistic is χ^2 with one degree of freedom. The test is highly significant, $P < 0.001$.

Furthermore, the test statistic for departures from a linear regression is $X_2^2 = X - X_1^2 = 19.28 - 19.27 = 0.01$ whose sampling distribution is χ^2 with one degree of freedom. This test is not significant, $P > 0.05$.

Thus it would appear that there is a definite linear trend in the proportions of children having a detectable measles haemagglutination inhibitory titre of less than 5, these proportions decreasing with the older age-at-vaccination categories.

Chapter 11
Linear Regression and Correlation

Linear relationships between two variables

The simplest situation concerns *two* quantitative variables x and y. For every value of x on an individual there is a corresponding value of y. It is assumed that the relationship between x and y is *linear*. Two problems are considered:

1. REGRESSION: Attention is centred on the *dependence* of one variable, y, on the other variable, x. An equation is determined which expresses this dependence mathematically. The statistical properties of the equation are investigated for purposes of prediction, estimation and hypothesis testing.

2. CORRELATION: Attention is centred on the *interdependence* between x and y which is quantified by a coefficient amenable to the techniques of statistical inference.

Diagrams

The first stage in the study of the relationship between the variables x and y should be a plot of the data to give an indication of the form and strength of the relationship. The random sample of n pairs of observations (x_1, y_1), (x_2, y_2), . . . , (x_n, y_n) is generally plotted on a rectangular coordinate system to obtain a *scatter diagram*. Conventionally, the horizontal axis corresponds to values of x and the vertical axis to values of y. From the scatter diagram it is often possible to visualise a smooth curve approximating the data—the *approximating curve*. A *linear* relationship exists if the approximating curve is a straight line.

Linear regression

Determination of the line

The straight line which best describes the relationship between the two variables x and y in the *population* is of the form

$$E(y|x) = \alpha + \beta x$$

Terminology

y: The *dependent* variable, a random variable.

x: The *independent*, predictor, prognostic or explanatory variable, assumed capable of measurement without error and used as a tool in the *prediction* of *y*. The regression line with *y* as the dependent variable and *x* as the independent variable is described as *the regression of y on x.*

$E(y|x)$: The expected value (mean) of *y* for a given *x*.

α: A parameter called the *intercept* of the line. It is the value of *y* (the ordinate) when $x = 0$.

β: A parameter called the *regression coefficient* or the gradient which measures the slope of the line, i.e. the change in *y* per unit increase in *x*.

α and β are the parameters which characterise a particular linear relationship.

Estimation of the parameters α and β

The problem of fitting a line to a sample of points is essentially the problem of efficiently estimating the parameters α and β (by *a* and *b*, respectively). The best known method for doing this is called the *method of least squares*. Since the fitted line is used for estimating or predicting values of *y* for specified values of *x*, a reasonable requirement is that the statistics *a* and *b* characterising the line be determined such that the *errors* of estimation are small. For a given value of *x*, the error of estimation is the difference between the observed value of *y* and the corresponding value of *y* obtained from the fitted line, i.e. for *i*th point (x_i, y_i) $(i = 1, 2, \ldots, n)$, the error of estimation is the difference $e_i = y_i - (a + bx_i)$ (see Fig. 11.1). These differences may be positive, negative or zero, although their signs are ignored in Fig. 11.1. At this juncture, *a* and *b* are unknown. A criterion which allows an optimal evaluation of *a* and *b* is to fit the line to the sample of *n* points so that the sum of the squared errors of estimation (residual sum of squares) is a minimum, i.e.

$$S = e_1^2 + e_2^2 + \ldots + e_n^2 = \sum_{i=1}^{n} [y_i - (a + bx_i)]^2$$

is a minimum. This is the method of least squares.

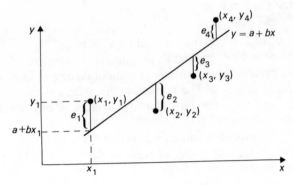

Fig. 11.1 Errors of estimation (e_i) for the fitted line $y = a+bx$.

Note

1. The *errors* are squared to overcome the nullifying effect of their opposing signs.

2. The random variable whose *i*th value is $\varepsilon_i = y_i-(\alpha+\beta x_i)$ is sometimes called the *residual* error or the residual. Rather unsatisfactorily, the difference $e_i = y_i-(a+bx_i)$ is also called the residual error or the residual.

3. The *distinction* between the independent (x) and the dependent (y) variables is important. The parameters defining the regression lines are different for the regression of y on x (giving consideration to the errors relative to y) and the regression of x on y (giving consideration to the errors relative to x) unless all the points of the scatter diagram lie on the line.

The minimisation of S, achieved by a mathematical technique called differentiation, produces the sample statistics a and b defined below, estimating the parameters α and β, respectively. The *estimated regression line* is then

$$y = a+bx$$

where

$$y = \bar{y}-b\bar{x}$$
$$b = S_{xy}/S_{xx}$$

where
    Sample mean of x:

$$\bar{x} = \sum x_i/n.$$

Sample mean of y:

$$\bar{y} = \sum y_i/n.$$

Corrected sum of squares of x:

$$S_{xx} = \sum (x_i - \bar{x})^2 = \sum x_i^2 - (\sum x_i)^2/n.$$

Corrected sum of squares of y:

$$S_{yy} = \sum (y_i - \bar{y})^2 = \sum y_i^2 - (\sum y_i)^2/n.$$

Corrected sum of products:

$$S_{xy} = \sum (x_i - \bar{x})(y_i - \bar{y}) = \sum x_i y_i - (\sum x_i)(\sum y_i)/n.$$

Using the estimated regression line

Linear regression analysis is performed to: (i) make inferences about the intercept, α; (ii) make inferences about the slope, β; (iii) predict the value of y for a given value of x; and (iv) identify unusual cases.

Assumptions

1. The values of x are observed without error.
2. For each value of x there is a *normal* distribution of values of y from which the observed sample value of y is drawn at random (see Fig. 11.2).

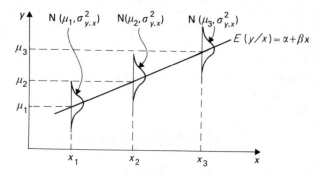

Fig. 11.2 Representation of the true linear regression line $E(y|x) = \alpha + \beta x$. The normal distribution of y about the regression line is shown for selected values of x.

3. The true *mean* value of the distribution of y for every value of x [$E(y|x) = \mu$] lies on a *straight* line which is the true regression line (see Fig. 11.2).

4. The *variance* (residual variance) of this normal distribution of values of y for a given value of x is constant for all values of x and equal to $\sigma_{y.x}^2$ (this property is called *homoscedasticity*) (see Fig. 11.2).

5. The observations (the y's) on different individuals can be adequately represented by mutually *independent* random variables.

These assumptions can be combined in either of the following statements: (i) each y_i is an independent observation drawn at random from the distribution $N(\alpha+\beta x_i, \sigma_{y.x}^2)$; or (ii) each error term, $\varepsilon_i = y_i - (\alpha + \beta x_i)$, is an independent deviation drawn at random from the distribution $N(0, \sigma_{y.x}^2)$. This error is independent of x.

The assumptions may also be checked by a graphical study of the residuals, $e_i = y_i - (a + bx_i)$, as described at the end of this chapter.

Estimation of $\sigma_{y.x}^2$

$\sigma_{y.x}^2$ is best estimated in the sample by

$$s_{y.x}^2 = \frac{1}{n-2}\left(S_{yy} - \frac{S_{xy}^2}{S_{xx}}\right) = \frac{1}{n-2}\sum_{}^{n}[y_i - (a + bx_i)]^2.$$

$s_{y.x}^2$ is an average (the divisor is $n-2$ instead of n to overcome bias) of the squared errors of estimation ($e_1^2, e_2^2, \ldots, e_n^2$) whose sum is minimised to determine a and b according to the method of least squares.

Intercept, α

1. *Properties of the sampling distribution of* $a = \bar{y} - b\bar{x}$.

    a. Normal.

    b. Mean $= \alpha$.

    c. Variance $= \sigma_a^2 = \sigma_{y.x}^2\left(\dfrac{1}{n} + \dfrac{\bar{x}^2}{S_{xx}}\right)$ estimated in the sample by

$$s_a^2 = s_{y.x}^2\left(\frac{1}{n} + \frac{\bar{x}^2}{S_{xx}}\right).$$

2. *Confidence interval for* α $(\sigma^2_{y.x}$ *unknown*).
Analogue: Confidence interval for μ; σ^2 unknown (Chapter 6).
The 95% confidence interval for α is

$$[a - t_{n-2}(0.025)s_a, \; a + t_{n-2}(0.025)s_a].$$

3. *Hypothesis test of* $\alpha(\sigma^2_{y.x}$ *unknown*).
Analogue: H_0: $\mu = \mu_0$; σ^2 unknown (Chapter 7).
   a. Define H_0: $\alpha = \alpha_0$. where α_0 is a particular value.
   b. Define H_1: $\alpha \neq \alpha_0$, say.
   c. Select a random sample of n pairs of observations (x_1, y_1), (x_2, y_2), . . . , (x_n, y_n).
   d. Draw a scatter diagram of the sample observations. Observe the form of the relationship, if any, between x and y; in particular, observe the value of the intercept of the regression line as judged by eye.
   e. Consider the test statistic, $T_{12} = (a - \alpha_0)/s_a$, whose sampling distribution is t on $n-2$ degrees of freedom.
   f. Compute the sample value, T_{12C}, of the test statistic from the sample data.
   g. Determine the critical region from tables of the t-distribution (Table A3). For a two-tailed test at the $200\alpha\%$ level of significance, reject H_0 if $|T_{12C}| > t_{n-2}(\alpha)$, $P < 2\alpha$. Do not reject H_0 otherwise, $P > 2\alpha$.

Slope, β

1. *Properties of the sampling distribution of* $b = S_{xy}/S_{xx}$.
   a. Normal.
   b. Mean $= \beta$.

   c. Variance $= \sigma^2_b = \dfrac{\sigma^2_{y.x}}{S_{xx}}$ estimated in the sample by

$$s^2_b = \frac{s^2_{y.x}}{S_{xx}}.$$

2. *Confidence interval for* β $(\sigma^2_{y.x}$ *unknown*).
Analogue: Confidence interval for μ; σ^2 unknown (Chapter 6).
The 95% confidence interval for β is

$$[b - t_{n-2}(0.025)s_b, \; b + t_{n-2}(0.025)s_b].$$

3. *Hypothesis test of* β *($\sigma_{y.x}^2$ unknown)*

Analogue: H_0: $\mu = \mu_0$; σ^2 unknown (Chapter 7).

    a. Define H_0: $\beta = \beta_0$, where β_0 is a particular value.

    b. Define H_1: $\beta \neq \beta_0$, say.

    c. Select a random sample of n pairs of observations (x_1, y_1), (x_2, y_2), . . . , (x_n, y_n).

    d. Draw a scatter diagram of the sample observations. Observe the form of the relationship, if any, between x and y; in particular, note whether a trend in any one direction is apparent.

    e. Consider the test statistic, $T_{13} = (b - \beta_0)/s_b$, whose sampling distribution is t on $n-2$ degrees of freedom.

    f. Compute the sample value, T_{13C}, of the test statistic from the sample data.

    g. Determine the critical region from tables of the t-distribution (Table A3). For a two-tailed test at the $200\alpha\%$ level of significance, reject H_0 if $|T_{13C}| > t_{n-2}(\alpha)$, $P < 2\alpha$. Do not reject H_0 otherwise, $P > 2\alpha$.

4. *Hypothesis test of the difference between two regression slopes,* β_1, β_2.

Analogue: H_0: $\mu_1 = \mu_2$; $\sigma_1^2 = \sigma_2^2 = \sigma^2$ unknown (Chapter 8).

    It is often of interest to determine whether the linear relationship between two variables x and y is the same in two populations; in particular, whether the slopes, β_1 and β_2, of the lines $E(y|x) = \alpha_1 + \beta_1 x$ and $E(y|x) = \alpha_2 + \beta_2 x$ are the same.

    a. Define H_0: $\beta_1 = \beta_2$.

    b. Define H_1: $\beta_1 \neq \beta_2$, say.

    c. Select a random sample of n_1 pairs of observations, (x_{11}, y_{11}), (x_{12}, y_{12}), . . . , (x_{1n_1}, y_{1n_1}), from the first population and an independent random sample of n_2 pairs of observations, (x_{21}, y_{21}), (x_{22}, y_{22}), . . . , (x_{2n_2}, y_{2n_2}), from the second population.

    d. Draw a scatter diagram of the two sets of points, distinguishing the two samples by different symbols or colours. Observe the form of the relationship, if any, between x and y in each set and note any obvious differences between the sets.

    e. Consider the test statistic

$$T_{14} = \frac{b_1 - b_2}{s_{b_1 - b_2}}$$

where, for $i = 1, 2$,

$$S_{xx_i} = \sum_{j}^{n_i} (x_{ij} - \overline{x}_i)^2$$

$$S_{yy_i} = \sum_{j}^{n_i} (y_{ij}-\bar{y}_i)^2$$

$$S_{xy_i} = \sum_{j}^{n_i} (x_{ij}-\bar{x}_i)(y_{ij}-\bar{y}_i)$$

$$s^2_{y.x_i} = \frac{1}{n_i-2}\left(S_{yy_i}-\frac{S^2_{xy_i}}{S_{xx_i}}\right)$$

and

$$b_1 = S_{xy_1}/S_{xx_1}$$

$$b_2 = S_{xy_2}/S_{xx_2}$$

$$s^2_{b_1-b_2} = s^2\left(\frac{1}{S_{xx_1}}+\frac{1}{S_{xx_2}}\right)$$

where

$$s^2 = \frac{(n_1-2)s^2_{y.x_1}+(n_2-2)s^2_{y.x_2}}{n_1+n_2-4}$$

The sampling distribution of T_{14} is t on n_1+n_2-4 degrees of freedom. This test statistic is chosen because:

(i) The difference between two regression coefficients, $\beta_1-\beta_2$, is estimated by the difference in their sample estimators, b_1-b_2.

(ii) The sampling distribution of b_i ($i = 1, 2$) is $N(\beta_i, \sigma^2_{y.x_i}/S_{xx_i})$. Hence the sampling distribution of b_1-b_2 is $N(\beta_1-\beta_2, \sigma^2_{y.x_1}/S_{xx_1}+\sigma^2_{y.x_2}/S_{xx_2})$.

(iii) The sampling distribution of

$$[(b_1-b_2)-(\beta_1-\beta_2)]\bigg/ \sqrt{\frac{\sigma^2_{y.x_1}}{S_{xx_1}}+\frac{\sigma^2_{y.x_2}}{S_{xx_2}}}$$

is standard normal. However, since $\sigma^2_{y.x_1}$ and $\sigma^2_{y.x_2}$ are rarely known in practice, they are replaced by their sample estimates $s^2_{y.x_1}$ and $s^2_{y.x_2}$, respectively. A pooled estimate may be obtained as a weighted sum of the two estimated variances, i.e. s^2, defined above. The sampling distribution of this modified test statistic

$$[(b_1-b_2)-(\beta_1-\beta_2)]/\sqrt{s^2(1/S_{xx_1}+1/S_{xx_2})}$$

is t on n_1+n_2-4 degrees of freedom, which has tabulated percentage points.

(iv) The parameter specification of H_0 is $\beta_1 - \beta_2 = 0$.

f. Compute the sample value, T_{14C}, of the test statistic from the sample data.

g. Determine the critical region from tables of the t-distribution (Table A3). For a two-tailed test at the $200\alpha\%$ level of significance, reject H_0 if $|T_{14C}| > t_{n_1+n_2-4}(\alpha)$, $P < 2\alpha$. Do not reject H_0 otherwise, $P > 2\alpha$.

COMMON SLOPE

If the slopes are not significantly different from each other, a common value, β, may be assumed for the regression slope in the two groups. This common slope is estimated in the sample by

$$b = \frac{S_{xy_1} + S_{xy_2}}{S_{xx_1} + S_{xx_2}}$$

with a variance estimated as

$$s_b^2 = \frac{s^2}{S_{xx_1} + S_{xx_2}}.$$

Prediction of the dependent variable, *y*

The estimated regression line, $y = a + bx$, may be used to predict y for a given value of x. Two situations must be distinguished:

1. *Prediction of an individual value of y for a new member of the population whose value of the independent variable is $x = x_0$, say.*

This is the most common situation.

a. Predicted value, y_0.

$$y_0 = a + bx_0.$$

b. Variance of y_0, $\sigma_{y_0}^2$.

$$\sigma_{y_0}^2 = \sigma_{y.x}^2 \left[1 + \frac{1}{n} + \frac{(x_0 - \bar{x})^2}{S_{xx}} \right].$$

estimated by

$$s_{y_0}^2 = s_{y.x}^2 \left[1 + \frac{1}{n} + \frac{(x_0 - \bar{x})^2}{S_{xx}} \right].$$

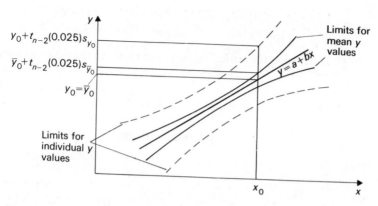

Fig. 11.3 95% confidence belts around the estimated regression line $y = a+bx$.

c. 95% confidence limits for the true value of y when $x = x_0$.

$$y_0 \pm t_{n-2}(0.025)s_{y_0}.$$

If calculations like this are done for various values of x and if the confidence limits are plotted above and below the estimated regression line, a confidence belt with curved borders is obtained (see Fig. 11.3). The belt contains the true value of y for a given value of x with 95% confidence.

2. *Prediction of the mean value of y when the value of the independent variable is $x = x_0$, say.*

a. Predicted mean value, $\bar{y}_0$.

$$\bar{y}_0 = a+bx_0 = y_0.$$

b. Variance of $\bar{y}_0$, $\sigma_{\bar{y}_0}^2$.

$$\sigma_{\bar{y}_0}^2 = \sigma_{y.x}^2 \left[\frac{1}{n} + \frac{(x_0-\bar{x})^2}{S_{xx}} \right]$$

estimated by

$$s_{\bar{y}_0}^2 = s_{y.x}^2 \left[\frac{1}{n} + \frac{(x_0-\bar{x})^2}{S_{xx}} \right].$$

c. 95% confidence limits for the true mean value of y when $x = x_0$.

$$\bar{y}_0 \pm t_{n-2}(0.025)s_{\bar{y}_0}.$$

A confidence belt with curved borders may be obtained by considering the confidence limits for different values of x (see Fig. 11.3). The belt provides a confidence region for the regression line, $E(y|x) = \alpha + \beta x$.

Linear correlation

The correlation coefficient

This relates to the *interdependence* (co-relation) between the two variables x and y. A measure of the degree of closeness of the linear relationship between the two variables is given by the (product moment) correlation coefficient, ρ. If a random sample of n pairs of observations is taken, $(x_1y_1), (x_2y_2), \ldots, (x_ny_n)$, ρ is estimated by the sample statistic r, where

$$r = \frac{\sum(x_i - \bar{x})(y_i - \bar{y})}{\sqrt{[\sum(x_i - \bar{x})^2 \sum(y_i - \bar{y})^2]}} = \frac{S_{xy}}{\sqrt{(S_{xx}S_{yy})}}.$$

Properties of r

1. $-1 \leqslant r \leqslant +1$.

2. *Magnitude* of r indicates the strength of the linear relationship between x and y.

    a. $r = 0$ indicates no linear relationship: there may be a non-linear relationship.

    b. $r = \pm 1$ indicates perfect correlation: all the points lie on the line.

3. *Sign* of r indicates whether y tends to increase (positive r) or decrease (negative r) with x.

4. Dimensionless.

5. *Sampling distribution* of r is not normal. The sampling distribution of $z = \frac{1}{2} \log_e [(1+r)/(1-r)]$ is approximately $N(\mu_z, \sigma_z^2)$ where $\mu_z = \frac{1}{2} \log_e [(1+\rho)/(1-\rho)]$ and $\sigma_z^2 = 1/(n-3)$. (*Note:* $\log_e$ may be written ln.) This transformation of r is called Fisher's z transformation.

6. *Interpretation* of r is devoid of any cause and effect implications.

7. r^2 is the proportion of the total variance of y that can be explained by the linear regression of y on x (or x on y); $(1-r^2)$ is the proportion unexplained by the regression (i.e. if the total variance of y estimated in the sample is $s_y^2 = S_{yy}/(n-1)$, then it can be shown that $1-r^2 \simeq s_{y.x}^2/s_y^2$.

8. $r = b\sqrt{S_{xx}/S_{yy}}$, where b is the estimated regression coefficient in $y = a+bx$.

Interpretation of r

Figure 11.4 illustrates the nature of r in different circumstances. Figure 11.4(a) $r = +1$: perfect positive correlation. As x increases, y increases. All points lie on the line. Figure 11.4(b) $r = -1$: perfect negative correlation. As x increases, y decreases. All points lie on the line. Figure 11.4(c) $0 < r < 1$: some degree of positive correlation. As x increases, there is a tendency for y to increase. Not all points lie on the line. Figure 11.4(d) $-1 < r < 0$: some degree of negative correlation. As x increases, there is a tendency for y to decrease. Not all points lie on the line. Figure 11.4(e) $r = 0$: no correlation. Figure 11.4(f) $r = 0$: no linear correlation, although the variables exhibit a non-linear relationship.

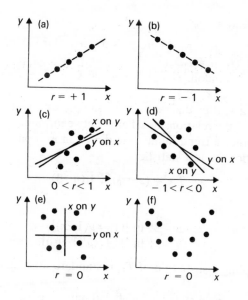

Fig. 11.4 Scatter diagrams with correlation coefficients ranging from -1 to $+1$. See text for fuller description.

Inferences concerning the correlation coefficient

The n pairs of observations (x_1, y_1), (x_2, y_2), . . . , (x_n, y_n) can be thought of as a random sample from a population of all such pairs. Since two variables are involved, this is called a *bivariate* population which is assumed to have a *bivariate normal distribution*.

Hypothesis test: H_0: $\rho = 0$

It can be shown that the test of H_0: $\rho = 0$ is equivalent to the test of H_0: $\beta = 0$ where β is the regression coefficient in $E(y|x) = \alpha + \beta x$. (*Note:* $r = b\sqrt{S_{xx}/S_{yy}}$ which implies that if $b = 0$ then $r = 0$. The test of H_0: $\beta = \beta_0$ (here $\beta_0 = 0$) is discussed under linear regression in Chapter 11.) As this test is performed often, special tables (Table A5) facilitate the answer (*note:* this test requires only that one variable be normally distributed; it makes no assumption that the pairs of observations in the sample come from a bivariate normal distribution).

Hypothesis test: H_0: $\rho = \rho_0 \neq 0$

1. Define H_0: $\rho = \rho_0$, where ρ_0 is a particular value.
2. Define H_1: $\rho \neq \rho_0$, say.
3. Select a random sample of n pairs of observations (x_1, y_1), (x_2, y_2), . . . , (x_n, y_n).
4. Draw a scatter diagram of the sample observations. Observe the form of the relationship, if any, between x and y; in particular, note whether a trend in any one direction is apparent.
5. Consider the test statistic

$$T_{15} = (z - z_0)/\sqrt{1/(n-3)}$$

where

$$z = \tfrac{1}{2} \ln [(1+r)/(1-r)]$$
$$z_0 = \tfrac{1}{2} \ln [(1+\rho_0)/(1-\rho_0)].$$

The sampling distribution of T_{15} is standard normal. T_{15} is chosen because:
    a. The sample statistic which estimates ρ is r.
    b. The sampling distribution of r is not normal but utilising Fisher's z transformation, the distribution of

$$z = \tfrac{1}{2} \ln [(1+r)/(1-r)]$$

is approximately $N(\mu_z, \sigma_z^2)$ where

$$\mu_z = \tfrac{1}{2} \ln [(1+\rho)/(1-\rho)] \quad \text{and} \quad \sigma_z^2 = 1/(n-3).$$

c. The sampling distribution of $(z-\mu_z)/\sigma_z$ is approximately standard normal which has tabulated percentage points.

d. The parameter specification of H_0 is $\rho = \rho_0$ or, equivalently, $\mu_z = z_0$.

6. Compute the value, T_{15C}, of the test statistic from the sample data.

7. Determine the critical region from tables of the standard normal distribution (Table A1). For a two-tailed test at the $200\alpha\%$ level of significance, reject H_0 if $|T_{15C}| > Z(\alpha)$, $P < 2\alpha$. Do not reject H_0 otherwise, $P > 2\alpha$.

95% confidence interval for ρ

The confidence interval for ρ is obtained from the confidence interval for μ_z by reversing the identity

$$\mu_z = \tfrac{1}{2} \ln [(1+\rho)/(1-\rho)]$$

so that

$$\rho = [\exp(2\mu_z)-1]/[\exp(2\mu_z)+1].$$

Since the sampling distribution of z is approximately $N[\mu_z, 1/(n-3)]$, the 95% confidence interval for μ_z is

$$\left[\tfrac{1}{2} \ln\left(\frac{1+r}{1-r}\right) - 1.96 \frac{1}{\sqrt{(n-3)}}, \ \tfrac{1}{2} \ln\left(\frac{1+r}{1-r}\right) + 1.96 \frac{1}{\sqrt{(n-3)}} \right]$$

where 1.96 is the appropriate percentage point of the standard normal distribution.

Hypothesis test of the difference between two correlation coefficients, ρ_1, ρ_2

Analogue: H_0: $\mu_1 = \mu_2$; σ_1^2, σ_2^2 known (Chapter 8).

1. Define H_0: $\rho_1 = \rho_2$.

2. Define H_1: $\rho_1 \neq \rho_2$.

3. Select a random sample of n_1 pairs of observations, (x_{11}, y_{11}), (x_{12}, y_{12}), . . . , (x_{1n_1}, y_{1n_1}), from the first population and an independent random sample of n_2 pairs of observations, (x_{21}, y_{21}), (x_{22}, y_{22}), . . . , (x_{2n_2}, y_{2n_2}), from the second population.

4. Draw a scatter diagram of the two sets of points, distinguishing the samples by different symbols or colours. Observe the form of the relationship, if any, between x and y in each set and note any obvious differences between sets.

5. Consider the test statistic

$$T_{16} = (z_1 - z_2)/\sqrt{1/(n_1 - 3) + 1/(n_2 - 3)}$$

where r_i is the estimated correlation coefficient from the ith sample ($i = 1, 2$) and

$$z_i = \tfrac{1}{2} \ln\left(\frac{1 + r_i}{1 - r_i}\right); i = 1, 2.$$

The sampling distribution of T_{16} is approximately standard normal.

6. Compute the value, T_{16C}, of the test statistic from the sample data.

7. Determine the critical region from tables of the standard normal distribution (Table A1). For a two-tailed test at the $200\alpha\%$ level of significance, reject H_0 if $|T_{16C}| > Z(\alpha)$, $P < 2\alpha$. Do not reject H_0 otherwise, $P > 2\alpha$.

Extensions of simple linear regression and correlation

The fundamental principles of simple linear regression and correlation involving two variables x and y may be extended to:

1. Multiple linear regression

This examines the linear relationship between a dependent variable, y, and two or more (not necessarily uncorrelated) independent, predictor, prognostic or explanatory variables, x_1, $x_2, \ldots$, by determining an equation which best (e.g. by the method of least squares) describes the relationship. For example, if there are two independent variables, the equation is of the form

$$E(y|x) = \alpha + \beta_1 x_1 + \beta_2 x_2,$$

estimated from the sample by

$$y = a + b_1 x_1 + b_2 x_2$$

and a plane in three-dimensional space may be fitted to the data points. The constant term, α, is sometimes called the *intercept*. The constants β_1 and β_2 are called *partial regression coefficients*. The coefficient β_1 measures the average change in y when x_1

changes by one unit, and x_2 (and any other x's for more extensive models) remains constant. It differs from the coefficient which would be obtained if some or all other independent variables were ignored and a simple regression of y on the one independent variable calculated.

The number of independent variables, k, should be substantially less than the number of individuals, n, from whom the data are collected, and information should be available on all variables for each individual.

Purposes

The main *purposes* of multiple regression are:

a. To discover which of the independent variables are related to y as an aid to understanding and perhaps controlling the response variable and, if possible, to discern the order of importance of these independent variables.

b. To predict values of y from the optimal equation relating y and the x's. When there are many x's it may be necessary to determine that subset of them which gives the best linear prediction equation.

Statistical analysis

Statistical methods, together with extensive computer programs, are available for estimating the intercept, α, and the partial regression coefficients, β_1, β_2, β_3, . . . , β_k, with their standard errors, and for making relevant inferences. In particular, typical *analyses* are:

a. An *F-test*, derived from an analysis of variance, to evaluate the significance of the joint relationship of y with the independent variables. It tests the null hypothesis that all the partial regression coefficients are zero. This test is equivalent to that of the significance of the multiple correlation coefficient (defined on p. 150) from zero.

b. A *t-test* to evaluate the significance of each partial regression coefficient, $\beta_i (i = 1, 2, . . . , k)$, from zero. The test statistic for H_0: $\beta_i = 0$ is the ratio of the estimated coefficients, b_i, to its estimated standard error. This has a t-distribution with $n - k - 1$ degrees of freedom, where n is the number of individuals. If the coefficient does not differ significantly from zero, the relevant independent variable may be omitted from the regression equation without any significant effect on the variation of y, and new coefficients estimated for the remaining x's.

c. An *analysis of variance* to test whether the variability of y is significantly affected by deletion of a group of predictor variables. Computer programs are generally available for the selection of an optimal set of independent variables.

d. *Automatic elimination procedures* to select the 'best' subset of independent variables. There is no unique statistical procedure for doing this. The main approaches include step-up, step-down and optimal combination procedures.

The reader is referred to Draper, N. R. and Smith, H. (1981) for a full discussion of the methods.

2. Multiple linear correlation

This examines the degree of the linear relationship between three or more variables. A distinction is drawn between the:

a. *Zero-order correlation coefficient*—the simple linear correlation coefficient which measures the degree of linear association between any two of the variables (e.g. ρ_{12}, the correlation coefficient between x_1 and x_2), ignoring the other variable(s).

b. *Partial correlation coefficient* which quantifies the linear correlation between any two of the variables in a cross-section of individuals whose values for each of the remaining variables are the same (e.g. $\rho_{12.3}$, the partial correlation coefficient between variables x_1 and x_2 in a cross-section of individuals all having the same value of x_3).

c. *Multiple correlation coefficient*—the product moment correlation coefficient between the actual values of the *dependent* variable and the values as given by the fitted regression equation. The coefficient is usually denoted by R in the sample, its square, R^2 (analogous to r^2 in simple linear regression), representing the proportion of the total variation of y explained by the multiple regression equation.

3. Polynomial regression

This examines the *non-linear* relationship between the dependent variable and one or more independent variables, e.g. the polynomial regression of y on one independent variable x may be:

Quadratic: $E(y|x) = \alpha + \beta_1 x + \beta_2 x^2$
Cubic: $E(y|x) = \alpha' + \beta_1' x + \beta_2' x^2 + \beta_3' x^3$
etc.

Polynomial regression may be thought of as a special case of multiple regression. For example, if the two independent variables, x_1 and x_2, in a multiple regression equation are replaced by x and x^2, respectively, then the resulting equation is the quadratic equation defined above.

The reader is referred to Armitage, P. (1987) pp. 318–324, for example and further discussion of the techniques.

4. The analysis of variance

The analysis of variance is discussed more fully in Chapter 9 but some insight into its relationship with multiple regression is given here. In fact, the analysis of variance may be thought of as a particular form of multiple regression. It is concerned with analysing experimental data to evaluate the contribution of certain factors to the total variation of the variable under study. One approach is to define a theoretical model which is believed to describe the experimental situation. This model may be expressed in the form of a multiple regression equation (with its associated assumptions) in which the variable being studied (e.g. systolic blood pressure) is the dependent variable, y, and the factors believed to be associated with defined sources of variation (e.g. age, weight) are the independent variables $x_1, x_2, \ldots$. The intercept, α, and the true regression coefficients $\beta_1, \beta_2, \ldots$, are estimated by the statistics $a, b_1, b_2, \ldots$, such that for a set of n individuals, the sum of squared errors of estimation,

$$\sum_{i}^{n} [y_i-(a+b_1x_{1i}+b_2x_{2i}+ \ldots)]^2,$$

is a minimum (according to the method of least squares).

5. Analysis of covariance

The analysis of covariance is an extension of the analysis of variance for classified data (the classes typically corresponding to treatments) when, in addition to having knowledge of values of the response variable, y, information is available on one or more explanatory, prognostic or predictor variables, $x_2, x_3, \ldots x_k$, known or suspected to influence the value of the response variable. If the data were not classified an ordinary multiple regression analysis would establish the linear relationship between y and the x's. However, in the analysis of covariance, interest is centred on the joint effect on y of the classification and of the prognostic variables.

The analysis of covariance derives two important benefits from combining the features of analysis of variance and regression: (i) it is possible to throw light on the nature of treatment effects when adjustments are made for possible sources of bias resulting from the treatment groups differing in their mean values of some or all of the prognostic factors, (ii) the precision of estimates and tests used to compare treatment groups is increased by reducing the variation within groups.

A full discussion, with examples, is given by Armitage, P. (1987) pp. 282–295 and pp. 313–318.

Procedure

The easiest approach to the analysis of covariance is to formulate the model as a multiple linear regression equation. This approach, appropriate for a *quantitative response*, proposes an additive model of the form

$$E(y|x_1, x_2, \ldots, x_k) = \alpha + \beta_1 x_1 + \beta_2 x_2 + \ldots + \beta_k x_k \quad (11.1)$$

where one variable (x_1, say) is a *dummy variable* specifying treatment when there are two treatment groups (*note*: the model can be generalised when there are more than two treatment groups by introducing a series of dummy variables).

A dummy variable is an 'artificial' variable which can take two arbitrary values, typically 0 and 1. It is created to enable a qualitative (i.e. non-measurable) factor to be included in the regression analysis. The partial regression coefficient for the dummy variable provides a measure of the difference in the corrected means of y in the two groups categorised by the values of the dummy variable, after adjusting for prognostic factors.

Thus, in the proposed model specified above, one variable (x_1, say) is a dummy variable specifying treatment (e.g. $x_1 = 0$ for treatment A and $x_1 = 1$ for treatment B) and all other x's (x_2, $x_3, \ldots, x_k$) are prognostic variables which are either quantitative or qualitative [for which dummy variables or artificial numerical variables (e.g. one taking the scores 1 to 5 for social classes I to V) are created].

Various *assumptions* are implicit in the analysis of covariance model. For example, using the above definition of x_1, the model can be written as

$$E(y|x_2, x_3, \ldots, x_k) = \begin{cases} \alpha + \beta_2 x_2 + \beta_3 x_3 + \ldots + \beta_k x_k \text{ for group A} \\ \alpha + \beta_1 + \beta_2 x_2 + \beta_3 x_3 + \ldots + \beta_k x_k \text{ for group B} \end{cases}$$

which shows that the model asserts that the corresponding partial regression coefficients are the same in the two treatment groups (i.e. that there are no interactions between the treatment effect and the covariates). Note that the intercepts of these two groups differ by β_1 so testing that $\beta_1 = 0$ is equivalent to testing that the difference in the intercepts in the two treatment groups is zero.

The techniques of multiple linear regression analysis may be applied to the analysis of covariance model (11.1) and , fortunately, computer programs are readily available. The intercept, α, and the partial regression coefficients with their standard errors are estimated and a t-test of the significance of each coefficient from zero can be performed to test whether each variable contributes to the regression. *Of particular interest* is the partial regression coefficient, β_1, for the treatments. If β_1 is significantly different from zero this provides an indication that the treatments differ after adjusting for prognostic factors.

Note: An alternative, but not recommended, procedure for evaluating treatment differences when various prognostic factors are thought to influence response is to estimate the treatment effect for various subgroups of the data defined by these prognostic factors. Such an approach should be viewed with caution as the numbers may be small in each subgroup and the results may be difficult to interpret. However, an initial look at the base-line data to check that the treatment groups are comparable with respect to prognostic factors is always to be recommended. Randomisation (see pp. 191–195) should promote comparability provided the sample sizes are not too small.

6. Multiple logistic regression

When treatment differences are to be evaluated for a *qualitative* response variable, y (often a *binary* variable which can take one of two values, typically 0 and 1), and measurements are available on prognostic variables thought to influence response (say x_2, $x_3, \ldots, x_k$) then the analysis of the covariance model outlined above may be unrealistic. Instead, attention is focused on the relation between the probability of success, p (prob($y = 1$), say) and the variables $x_1, x_2, \ldots, x_k$, one of which (x_1, say) is a dummy variable representing treatment. Similarly, this type of relationship is useful when interest is centred solely on the effect of various prognostic variables on a binary response variable (i.e. in the absence of any treatment comparisons).

One of the simplest ways of representing the dependence of p on $x_1, x_2, \ldots, x_k$ so that the constraint $0 \leq p \leq 1$ is satisfied, is by considering the linear relationship

$$\log_e \frac{p}{1-p} = \alpha + \beta_1 x_1 + \beta_2 x_2 + \ldots + \beta_k x_k \qquad (11.2)$$

which is called the *multiple logistic model*. The quantity $p/(1-p)$ is equal to the *odds* in favour of success and $\log_e p/(1-p)$ is equal to the log odds (or *logit*). The coefficient β_1 is equal to the change in the log odds corresponding to a change of one unit in x_1, and hence to the log of the ratio of two odds. This means that $\exp(\beta_1)$ is an *odds ratio*. Similarly for $\beta_2, \ldots, \beta_k$.

Thus, if x_1 is a dummy variable representing treatment effect in the multiple logistic model, the odds ratio is $\exp(\beta_1)$; i.e. the odds of 'success' are $\exp(\beta_1)$ times higher in those with the treatment than those without it. Furthermore, the coefficients ($\beta_i; i = 2, 3, \ldots, k$) of the other variables ($x_i; i = 2, 3, \ldots, k$) each provide a measure of the effect of the associated variable on the outcome. For example, each additional unit of the quantitative variable x_2 (say) increases the log odds of 'success' by β_2 [or multiplies the odds of success by $\exp(\beta_2)$]. It should be noted that the value of α refers to a level rather than a difference and is not generally interpretable.

Computer programs are available for the relatively complex iterative procedure of estimating the coefficients in a logistic regression, with their standard errors. *t*-tests can be performed, as in multiple linear regression, to evaluate their significance. The reader is referred to Anderson, S. *et al.* (1980), pp. 161–177, for a full discussion.

Note: A simpler method of assessing the significance of a treatment difference after adjusting for just one or two qualitative prognostic factors when there is a binary response variable is to use the *Mantel–Haenszel test* (the log-rank test, suitable for survival data, is also sometimes called the Mantel–Haenszel test; see pp. 212–213). In the Mantel–Haenszel test, the data are presented as a series of fourfold tables, each of the form of Table 15.2, one for every classification of the prognostic variable(s). In this context, disease status (present or absent) is replaced by treatment (present or absent), and factor (present or absent) is replaced by outcome (success or failure). The test statistic, S^2 (defined on p. 232), is used to test the null hypothesis that there is no association between treatment and outcome (i.e. that treatment makes no difference to the probability of success), after adjusting for the prognostic variable(s).

7. Linear discriminant functions

Multiple regression theory can be used in linear discriminant analysis, one of the many techniques of *multivariate analysis* [i.e. the analysis of data from n (say) individuals on each of whom are observed the values of k (say) variables]. The problem in discriminant analysis is to determine a rule for discriminating between two or more populations. A sample of individuals (each individual having measurements on k variables, $x_1, x_2, \ldots, x_k$) is taken from each population. Ideally, the discriminating rule can be used to allocate further individuals, whose correct population of origin is unknown, to the correct population with minimal probability of misclassification.

Example

Suppose it is difficult to distinguish two diseases on the basis of signs and symptoms, and that only a biopsy involving surgical operation provides a definite diagnosis. Discriminant analysis, performed on a data set from cases in whom biopsy has made the diagnosis certain, may enable a future patient to be diagnosed without biopsy.

Rule

One rule for discriminating between two populations is obtained from the discriminant function derived from the multiple logistic regression equation [of the form of Equation (11.2) in the previous section] in which y is a dummy variable taking the value 0 for every individual in one population (A, say) and 1 for every individual in the other population (B, say), and p is the prob($y = 1|x_1$, $x_2, \ldots, x_k$). The values of logit p (often called the z-scores) from the fitted logistic regression equation (whose coefficients are estimated from the data available from the initial samples) should be less than 0 ($p < \frac{1}{2}$) for those individuals in population A and greater than 0 ($p > \frac{1}{2}$) for those in population B. The allocation to population A or B of a new individual, known to come from one of these populations (the particular population being unknown) will depend on his z-score, obtained from the fitted logistic regression equation, given his values of $x_1, x_2, \ldots, x_k$.

This approach is particularly useful when discrimination is required between two or more populations on the basis of discrete variables, possibly with some continuous variables as well. The reader is referred to Anderson, J. A. (1972) pp. 19–34 for a full discussion, including a practical illustration of the technique. Alternative approaches to determining a discriminant function are discussed by Armitage, P. (1987) pp. 326–347.

Validation of assumptions in regression analysis

The assumptions on which regression analysis is based are stated at the beginning of this chapter. Expressed concisely, the values of the residual error for different individuals are independently and normally distributed with zero mean and constant variance, $\sigma_{y.x}^2$. These assumptions are most easily validated and the form of the regression equation checked by a *graphical study of the residuals*. The residual error for the ith individual is the difference between the observed value, y_i, of the dependent variable for that individual and the corresponding predicted value obtained from the estimated (linear/multiple/polynomial) regression equation (e.g. in linear regression, the residual is $e_i = y_i - (a + bx_i)$ for the ith individual). Some potentially useful scatter diagrams are:

1. **Plot of the residual against the predicted value [e.g. e_i vs $(a + bx_i)$].**

Purpose: to check the distributional assumptions made about the residuals, in particular: (i) normality; and (ii) constant variance (homoscedasticity).

Remedy: non-normality and heteroscedasticity of residuals may sometimes be remedied by a transformation of the dependent variable (see Chapter 12).

2. **Plot of the residual against the value of the independent variable (e_i vs x_i).**

The residuals may be plotted against the values of any or all of the independent variables (there is one independent variable in linear regression; more than one in multiple linear regression).

Purpose: to check the form of the (multiple) linear regression equation. A non-linear trend suggests that a *linear* regression equation inadequately represents the effect of the independent variable.

Remedy: a simple solution might be to add a term of higher order {e.g. to change the form of the regression equation from linear $[E(y|x) = \alpha+\beta x]$ to quadratic $[E(y|x) = \alpha_0+\beta_1 x+\beta_2 x^2]$}.

3. Plot of the residual against the value of a new variable, x' (e_i vs x'_i).

Purpose: to check that sufficient independent variables are included in the regression equation. The presence of correlation in this plot (the residuals are uncorrelated with the predicted values of the dependent variable and with the values of the independent variables) indicates that perhaps this new variable which has not been included in the regression equation, should be included.

Remedy: include the new variable, x', in the regression equation as an additional independent variable.

Examples

Determination of the line

Table E11.1 shows the age and 6 hour postoperative measurements of Pa_{O_2} in a random sample of 10 patients who undergo varicose vein operations receiving 50% nitrous oxide with oxygen. Figure E11.1 shows the scatter of the sample values.

$$\bar{x} = 385/10 = 38.5$$
$$\bar{y} = 862/10 = 86.2$$
$$S_{xx} = \sum x^2-(\sum x)^2/n = 15573-(385)^2/10 = 750.5$$
$$S_{yy} = \sum y^2-(\sum y)^2/n = 74968-(862)^2/10 = 663.6$$
$$S_{xy} = \sum xy-(\sum x)(\sum y)/n = 32870-(385)(862)/10 = -317$$
$$n = 10.$$

$$b = S_{xy}/S_{xx} = (-317)/(750.5) = -0.422$$
$$a = \bar{y}-b\bar{x} = 86.2-(-0.422)(38.5) = 102.46$$

The estimated regression line is

$$y = 102.46-0.422x.$$

Using the estimated regression line

Estimation of $\sigma^2_{y.x}$

$$s^2_{y.x} = \frac{1}{n-2}\left(S_{yy} - \frac{S^2_{xy}}{S_{xx}}\right)$$
$$= \frac{1}{8}\left(663.6 - \frac{(-317)^2}{750.5}\right)$$
$$= 66.21.$$

Intercept

$$s^2_a = s^2_{y.x}\left(\frac{1}{n} + \frac{\bar{x}^2}{S_{xx}}\right)$$
$$= 66.21\left(\frac{1}{10} + \frac{(38.5)^2}{750.5}\right)$$
$$= 137.39$$
$$s_a = 11.72.$$

The intercept, α, is the value of the patient's 6 hour postoperative Pa_{O_2} (mm Hg) when his age (years) is zero. Clearly, in the present context, the intercept has little meaning, for attention is restricted to adults. Thus it is futile to attempt to evaluate confidence limits for α or to test an hypothesis of α.

Slope

$$s^2_b = s^2_{y.x}/S_{xx}$$
$$= (66.21)/(750.2)$$
$$= 0.088$$
$$s_b = 0.297.$$

Table E11.1 Age and 6 hour postoperative Pa_{O_2} in 10 patients receiving 50% nitrous oxide with oxygen during operation.

Patient	1	2	3	4	5	6	7	8	9	10
Age (years): x	47	26	34	36	24	45	39	37	44	53
Pa_{O_2} (mm Hg): y	74	91	78	99	94	76	95	82	86	87

Source: Wildsmith, J. A. W. and Masson, A. H. B. (1974), Some effects of maintaining nitrogenation during anaesthesia. *Br. J. Anaesth.* **46**, 680–684.

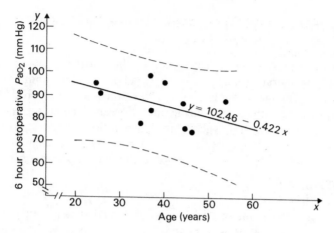

Fig. E11.1 Scatter diagram showing the 6 hour postoperative Pa_{O_2} and ages of 10 patients receiving 50% nitrous oxide with oxygen during operation. The estimated regression line and 95% confidence limits for the observations are shown. Source: Table E11.1.

CONFIDENCE INTERVAL FOR β ($\sigma^2_{y.x}$ UNKNOWN)

The 95% confidence interval for β is

$$(b - t_{n-2}(0.025)s_b, \; b + t_{n-2}(0.025)s_b)$$
$$= [-0.422 - (2.31)(0.297), \; -0.422 + (2.31)(0.297)]$$
$$= (-1.108, 0.264).$$

HYPOTHESIS TEST OF β ($\sigma^2_{y.x}$ UNKNOWN)

1. H_0: β = 0.
2. H_1: β ≠ 0.
3. A random sample of 10 patients is selected. Their ages and 6 hour postoperative Pa_{O_2} measurements are given in Table E11.1.
4. Figure E11.1 is a scatter diagram of the sample observations. There does not appear to be a linear relationship between x and y.
5. Consider $T_{13} = (b - \beta_0)/s_b$.
6. $T_{13C} = (-0.422 - 0)/(0.297)$
$$= -1.42.$$
7. From tables of the t-distribution, $t_8(0.025) = 2.31$. Hence $|T_{13C}| < t_8(0.025)$ since $1.42 < 2.31$. Thus do not reject H_0 that the slope of the regression line is zero, $P > 0.05$.

HYPOTHESIS TEST OF THE DIFFERENCE BETWEEN TWO REGRESSION COEFFICIENTS

It is of interest to investigate whether the linear regression of 6 hour postoperative $Pao_2(y)$ on age (x) in patients undergoing varicose vein operations is the same when the patients receive 50% nitrous oxide with oxygen during operation and when they receive 50% nitrogen with oxygen during operation. The regression equations are respectively, $E(y|x) = \alpha_1 + \beta_1 x$ (estimated by $y = a_1 + b_1 x$) and $E(y|x) = \alpha_2 + \beta_2 x$ (estimated by $y = a_2 + b_2 x$).

1. H_0: $\beta_1 = \beta_2$.
2. H_1: $\beta_1 \neq \beta_2$.
3. A random sample of 10 patients is selected. The patients have varicose vein operations receiving 50% nitrous oxide with oxygen. Their ages and 6 hour postoperative Pao_2 values are shown in Table E11.1. The linear regression line is estimated as $y = 102.46 - 0.422x$ ($S_{xx_1} = 750.5$, $S_{xy_1} = -317$, $s_{y.x_1}^2 = 66.21$, $n_1 = 10$). A second independent random sample of 10 patients have varicose vein operations receiving 50% nitrogen with oxygen during operation. The ages and 6 hour postoperative Pao_2 values for these patients are shown in Table E11.2. The linear regression line is estimated as $y = 123.51 - 1.150x$ ($S_{xx_2} = 305.60$, $S_{xy_2} = -3514$, $s_{y.x_2}^2 = 169.00$, $n_2 = 10$).

Table E11.2 Age and 6 hour postoperative Pao_2 in 10 patients receiving 50% nitrogen with oxygen during operation

Patient	11	12	13	14	15	16	17	18	19	20
Age (years): x	36	45	55	46	34	44	39	42	44	43
Pao_2 (mm Hg): y	85	81	74	49	90	64	90	75	79	56

Source: Wildsmith, J. A. W. and Masson, A. H. B. (1974), *Br. J. Anaesth.* **46**, 680–684.

4. Figure E11.2 is a scatter diagram of the two sets of sample observations. The two estimated regression lines are indicated in the figure. They do not appear to differ.
5. Consider

$$T_{14} = \frac{b_1 - b_2}{s_{b_1 - b_2}}.$$

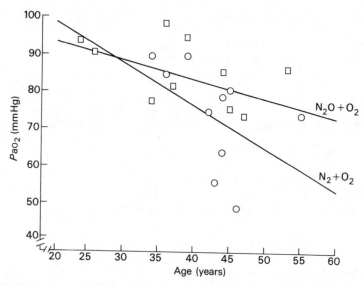

Fig. E11.2 Scatter diagram showing Pa_{O_2} and age in one sample of patients receiving 50% nitrous oxide ($\square$) and another sample of patients receiving 50% nitrogen with oxygen ($\bigcirc$). Estimated regression lines are drawn.

6.
$$
\begin{aligned}
s^2 &= [(n_1-2)s_{y.x_1}^2 + (n_2-2)s_{y.x_2}^2]/(n_1+n_2-4) \\
&= [8(66.21)+8(169.00)]/(10+10-4) \\
&= 117.605 \\
s_{b_1-b_2}^2 &= s^2(1/S_{xx_1}+1/S_{xx_2}) \\
&= 117.605[1/(750.50)+1/(305.60)] \\
&= 0.542 \\
s_{b_1-b_2} &= 0.736.
\end{aligned}
$$

Hence

$$
\begin{aligned}
T_{14C} &= [(-0.422)-(-1.150)]/(0.736) \\
&= 0.99.
\end{aligned}
$$

7. From tables of the t-distribution (Table A3), $t_{16}(0.025) = 2.12$. Hence $|T_{14C}| < t_{16}(0.025)$ since $0.99 < 2.12$. Thus do not reject H_0 that the slopes of the two regression lines are equal, $P > 0.05$.

Common slope

$$
\begin{aligned}
b &= (S_{xy_1}+S_{xy_2})/(S_{xx_1}+S_{xx_2}) \\
&= [(-317)+(-351.4)]/[750.50+305.60] \\
&= -0.633
\end{aligned}
$$

with a variance estimated as

$$s_b^2 = s^2/(S_{xx_1} + S_{xx_2})$$
$$= (117.605)/(750.50 + 305.60)$$
$$= 0.111.$$

Prediction of the dependent variable, y

PREDICTION OF AN INDIVIDUAL VALUE OF y

Consider the regression of 6 hour postoperative Pao_2 (mm Hg) on age (years) in the group of patients receiving 50% nitrous oxide with oxygen. The estimated regression line is

$$y = 102.46 - 0.422x$$
$$(s_{y.x}^2 = 66.21,\ S_{xx} = 750.5,\ \bar{x} = 38.5,\ n = 10).$$

The calculations leading to the determination of the 95% confidence limits for the true value of Pao_2 when the age takes different values are shown in Table E11.3. The confidence limits are plotted in Fig. E11.1.

Table E11.3 95% confidence limits for individual values of y (Pao_2) for various values of x (age)

Age (years) (x_0)	Corresponding Pao_2 (mm Hg) (y_0)	$s_{y_0} = \sqrt{s_{y.x}^2\left[1+\dfrac{1}{n}+\dfrac{(x_0-\bar{x})^2}{S_{xx}}\right]}$	95% confidence interval for y_0 when $t_8(0.025) = 2.31$	
			Lower limit $y_0 - 2.31 s_{y_0}$ (mm Hg)	Upper limit $y_0 + 2.31 s_{y_0}$ (mm Hg)
20	94.02	10.15	70.57	117.47
25	91.91	9.43	70.13	113.69
30	89.80	8.90	69.24	110.69
35	87.69	8.60	67.82	107.56
40	85.58	8.55	65.83	105.33
45	83.47	8.75	63.27	103.68
50	81.36	9.19	60.13	102.59
55	79.25	9.84	56.52	101.98

Source: Table E11.1.

Linear correlation coefficient

Suppose the correlation coefficient between 6 hour postoperative Pa_{O_2} (mm Hg) and age (years) in patients receiving nitrous oxide with oxygen during varicose vein operations is ρ. The sample product moment correlation coefficient from the data of Table E11.1 is

$$r = S_{xy}/\sqrt{S_{xx}S_{yy}}$$
$$= (-317)/\sqrt{(750.50)(663.60)}$$
$$= -0.45.$$

Inferences concerning the correlation coefficient

HYPOTHESIS TEST: H_0: $\rho = 0$

The Pa_{O_2} values (y) in the 10 patients are approximately normally distributed. The critical value of the sample correlation coefficient at the 5% level of significance is 0.63 (from Table A5, $v = n-2 = 8$). Since $|r| = 0.45 < 0.63$, do not reject H_0 that the true correlation coefficient is zero (equivalent to not rejecting H_0: $\beta = 0$, earlier), $P > 0.05$.

HYPOTHESIS TEST: H_0: $\rho = \rho_0 \neq 0$

1. H_0: $\rho = -0.9$.
2. H_1: $\rho \neq -0.9$.
3. A random sample of 10 patients is selected. Their ages and 6 hour postoperative Pa_{O_2} measurements are given in Table E11.1.
4. Figure E11.1 is a scatter diagram of the sample observations. Although there appears to be a trend (high values of x are associated with low values of y), it is not marked. It is assumed that the pairs of observations come from a bivariate normal distribution.
5. Consider

$$T_{15} = (z-z_0)/\sqrt{1/(n-3)}$$

where

$$z = \tfrac{1}{2}\log_e[(1+r)/(1-r)]$$
$$= \tfrac{1}{2}\log_e\{[1+(-0.45)]/[1-(-0.45)]\}$$
$$= -0.48$$
$$z_0 = \tfrac{1}{2}\log_e[(1+\rho_0)/(1-\rho_0)]$$
$$= \tfrac{1}{2}\log_e\{[1+(-0.9)]/[1-(-0.9)]\}$$
$$= -1.47$$

6. $T_{15C} = [(-0.48)-(-1.47)]/\sqrt{1/(10-3)}$
                       $= 2.62.$

7. From tables of the standard normal distribution (Table A1), $Z(0.025) = 1.96$, $Z(0.005) = 2.58$ and $Z(0.004) = 2.65$. Hence $|T_{15C}| > Z(0.005)$ since $2.62 > 2.58$ but $|T_{15C}| < Z(0.004)$ since $2.62 < 2.65$. Thus reject H_0 that the correlation coefficient is -0.9, $0.008 < P < 0.01$.

CONFIDENCE INTERVAL FOR ρ

The 95% confidence interval for

$$\mu_z = \tfrac{1}{2}\ln\left[(1+\rho)/(1-\rho)\right]$$

is

$$\left[\tfrac{1}{2}\ln\left(\frac{1+r}{1-r}\right)-1.96\sqrt{\frac{1}{n-3}},\ \tfrac{1}{2}\ln\left(\frac{1+r}{1-r}\right)+1.96\sqrt{\frac{1}{n-3}}\right]$$

$$= \left\{\tfrac{1}{2}\ln\left[\frac{1+(-0.45)}{1-(-0.45)}\right]-1.96\sqrt{\frac{1}{10-3}},\right.$$

$$\left.\tfrac{1}{2}\ln\left[\frac{1+(-0.45)}{1-(-0.45)}\right]+1.96\sqrt{\frac{1}{10-3}}\right\}$$

$$= (-0.48-0.74,\ -0.48+0.74)$$
$$= (-1.22,\ 0.26).$$

But

$$\rho = (\exp(2\mu_z)-1)/(\exp(2\mu_z)+1).$$

When $\mu_z = -1.22$,

$$\rho = \{\exp[2(-1.22)]-1\}/\{\exp[2(-1.22)]+1\}$$
$$= -0.84.$$

When $\mu_z = 0.26$,

$$\rho = \{\exp[2(0.26)]-1\}/\{\exp[2(0.26)]+1\}$$
$$= 0.25.$$

Hence the 95% confidence interval for ρ, assuming the pairs of observations come from a bivariate normal distribution, is $(-0.84, 0.25)$.

HYPOTHESIS TEST OF THE DIFFERENCE BETWEEN TWO CORRELATION COEFFICIENTS

The two correlation coefficients of interest are those which describe the linear relationships of the 6 hour postoperative Pao_2 measurement with age in patients undergoing varicose vein operations receiving either 50% nitrous oxide with oxygen (correlation coefficient ρ_1) or 50% nitrogen with oxygen (correlation coefficient ρ_2).

1. H_0: $\rho_1 = \rho_2$.
2. H_1: $\rho_1 \neq \rho_2$.
3. Two independent random samples, each of 10 patients, are selected. The data for these patients are shown in Tables E11.1 and E11.2. It is assumed that each of the samples contains pairs of observations from a bivariate normal distribution.
4. Figure E11.2 is a scatter diagram of the two sets of sample observations. The scatter of each set around its estimated regression line drawn in the diagram does not appear to be different for the two sets.
5. Consider $T_{16} = (z_1 - z_2)/\sqrt{1/(n_1 - 3) + 1/(n_2 - 3)}$.

6. a. Nitrous oxide:

$$r_1 = -0.45, \qquad z_1 = -0.48, \qquad n_1 = 10.$$

b. Nitrogen:

$$r_2 = (-351.4)/\sqrt{(305.60)(1756.10)} = -0.48$$
$$z_2 = \frac{1}{2} \ln[(1+r_2)/(1-r_2)] = -0.52$$
$$n_2 = 10.$$

Hence

$$T_{16C} = [(-0.48) - (-0.52)]/\sqrt{1/7 + 1/7}$$
$$= 0.07.$$

7. From tables of the standard normal distribution (Table A1), $Z(0.025) = 1.96$. Hence $|T_{16C}| < Z(0.025)$ since $0.07 < 1.96$. Thus do not reject H_0 that the correlation coefficients are equal, $P > 0.05$.

Chapter 11

Extensions of simple linear regression and correlation

Multiple linear regression

Mortality from coronary heart disease in civil servants in the lowest grade of employment has been found to be about three times that of men in the highest grade of employment. As part of an investigation of this finding several haemostatic variables were measured in a sample of 29 men in lower grades of employment and 45 men in higher grades (see Markowe, H. L. J., *et al*, 1985).

Previous studies have implicated fibrinogen (which tends to be log normally distributed) as a risk factor for cardiovascular disease. Consequently, a multiple regression analysis was performed with log fibrinogen concentration as the dependent variable. In addition to grade of employment, the independent variables were those characteristics previously shown to be significantly related to fibrinogen concentration: age, smoking, obesity [expressed as the body mass index, calculated as weight/(height)^2] and plasma total cholesterol concentration. The results are presented in Table E11.4.

The analysis showed significant associations of fibrinogen concentration with smoking ($P < 0.05$) and grade of employment ($P < 0.05$) after adjusting for the other variables. The multiple regression, including all the characteristics listed in Table E11.4, explained about 26% of the total variance in log fibrinogen concentration (i.e. $R^2 = 0.26$ where R is the estimated multiple correlation coefficient).

A simpler analysis of the data showed that the unadjusted difference in mean fibrinogen concentration between different grades of employment was large [3.39 (SD = 0.71) g/l in men in lower grades and 2.95 (SD = 0.50) g/l in men in higher grades, $P < 0.01$] but was not significant in other haemostatic variables.

The results of the study were thus consistent with a hypothesis that raised concentrations of fibrinogen could contribute to the increased mortality from coronary heart disease experienced by civil servants in low grades of employment.

Analysis of covariance

Cockburn, F., *et al* (1980) report the results of a clinical trial for prevention of infant hypocalcaemia in which 233 pregnant women

Table E11.4 Multiple regression of $\log_e$ (fibrinogen) in relation to other variables ($n = 74$)

i	Prognostic variable, x_i	Definition of x_i	Estimated partial regression coefficient (b_i)	Estimated standard error of b_i [SÊ(b_i)]	P value (H_0: $\beta_i = 0$) from t-test*
1	Age	years	0.006	0.004	0.10
2	Smoking	non-smoker = 0, smoker = 1	0.10	0.04	0.03
3	Body mass index	kg/m^2	0.012	0.009	0.17
4	Grade of employment	high = 0, low = 1	0.10	0.04	0.03
5	Plasma total cholesterol	mmol/l	0.024	0.021	0.24
	Estimated intercept with estimated SE		0.31	0.26	

Source: Markowe, H. L. J., Marmot, M. G., Shipley, M. J. *et al* (1985) Fibrinogen: a positive link between social class and coronary heart disease. *Br. Med. J.*, **291**, 1312–1314.

*For the ith prognostic variable ($i = 1, 2, \ldots, 5$), the test statistic is $b_i/[\text{SÊ}(b_i)]$ which has a t-distribution with $74-5-1 = 68$ degrees of freedom.

receiving vitamin D supplements were compared with a control group of 394 women receiving a placebo. The infant's plasma calcium concentration (mg per 100 ml) measured 6 days after birth was of principal interest and was chosen as the response variable, y. A dummy variable, x_1, was created for treatment such that $x_1 = 0$ for those in the control group and $x_1 = 1$ for those receiving vitamin D. The 10 prognostic variables were type of feed (artificial = 0, breast = 1), sex of infant (male = 0, female = 1), maternal age (years), total parity, social class (I to V scored 1 to 5), marital status (married = 0, unmarried = 1) birthweight (kg), gestational period (weeks), special care unit (not in SCU = 0, in SCU = 1) and pre-eclamptic toxaemia (no PET = 0, PET = 1).

A multiple regression analysis was performed using a suitable computer program. The regression coefficients for $x_1, x_2, \ldots, x_{11}$ were estimated, with their standard errors, and a t-test performed for each one. The results of the analysis are reported by Pocock, S. I. (1983), pp. 217–218, and summarised, together with the results of additional investigations, by Cockburn, F. *et al.* (1980). The regression coefficient for the dummy variable, x_1, representing treatment is of particular interest. It is 0.354 (standard error = 0.103, $t = 3.44$, $P < 0.001$). This indicates that the mean increase in plasma calcium using vitamin D, adjusting for prognostic factors, is estimated as 0.354 mg per 100 ml which is highly significant.

It is of interest to note that only two prognostic factors had regression coefficients significantly different from zero. They were sex (estimated coefficient = 0.256, standard error = 0.100, $P = 0.01$) and type of feed (estimated coefficient = 0.717, standard error = 0.115, $P < 0.001$). A further multiple regression analysis utilising only these two prognostic variables and the dummy variable representing treatment as the independent variables resulted in the infant's sixth-day plasma calcium concentration being predicted by the formula: 8.686+0.336 if mother given vitamin D +0.771 if breast-fed +0.254 if female, with a standard error of prediction of 1.220 mg per 100 ml. Thus the greatest influence on infant plasma calcium concentration was type of feed.

Multiple logistic regression

Walker, S. H. and Duncan, D. B. (1967) estimated a multiple

Table E11.5 Multiple logistic model for occurrence of CHD in the 5209 participants in the Framingham study

i	Prognostic variable, x_i	Definition of x_i	Estimated logistic coefficient, b_i	Test statistic t_i	Significance of t_i	Estimated relative risk, $\hat{R}_i$	95% confidence limits for relative risk, R_i
1	Sex	Male = 0, Female = 1	−1.5883	−9.12	$P < 0.001$	0.20	0.14 & 0.29
2	Age	years	0.0810	10.15	$P < 0.001$	1.08	1.07 & 1.10
3	Height	inches	−0.0528	−2.28	$0.02 < P < 0.05$	0.95	0.95 & 1.00
4	Systolic BP	mg Hg	0.0091	2.50	$0.01 < P < 0.02$	1.01	1.00 & 1.02
5	Diastolic BP	mg Hg	0.0055	0.81	$P > 0.05$	1.01	1.01 & 1.02
6	Serum cholesterol	mg per ml	0.0066	5.41	$P < 0.001$	1.01	1.00 & 1.01
7	ECG abnormalities	Absent = 0, Present = 1	0.8543	4.99	$P < 0.001$	2.35	1.67 & 3.31
8	Relative weight	Percentage, see note 1	1.3586	3.77	$P < 0.001$	3.89	1.89 & 8.00
9	Alcohol consumption	oz/month, see note 2	−0.0587	−1.60	$P > 0.05$	0.94	0.88 & 1.01
		Constant term, a = −5.3695					

Source: Walker, S. H. and Duncan, D. B. (1967) Estimation of the probability of an event as a function of several independent variables. *Biometrika*, **54**, 167–179.

Note 1: Relative weight = weight (lb) divided by median weight (lb) of sex-height group, as a percentage.

Note 2: Alcohol consumption coded as 0–6 for consumptions of 0, < 4, 5–14, 15–39, 40–69, 70–99, 100–999 oz/month in men, and coded as 0–5 for consumptions of 0, < 1, 1–9, 10–24, 25–39, 40–999 oz/month in women, respectively.

Note 3: The magnitude of the estimated relative risk, $\hat{R}_i$, is dependent on the scale of measurement of x_i.

logistic regression equation which determined the log odds of the probability of occurrence of coronary heart disease (CHD) as a function of nine independent variables. They analysed data from the Framingham study (Dawber, T. R., Meadors, G. F. and Moore, F. E., Jr., 1951) and some of their results are presented in Table E11.5. The response variable, y, was CHD coded as zero if absent and one if present, as determined by well-defined diagnostic criteria approximately 10 years from the date of determination of the values of the prognostic variables for the given individual.

Table E11.5 contains the estimated regression coefficients, b_i, and the values, t_i, of their sizes relative to their estimated standard errors. Each test statistic, t_i, is used to test the null hypothesis that the associated β_i, estimated by b_i, is zero by referring to the table of the t-distribution (Table A3) with ∞ (representing $5209 - 9 - 1 = 5199$) degrees of freedom (the approach used in multiple regression). Thus each test provides an evaluation of the importance of a particular prognostic variable, having adjusted for all other variables in the regression model.

From Table E11.5 it can be seen that age, systolic blood pressure, serum cholesterol, ECG abnormalities and relative weight have significant positive coefficients indicating that the log odds, and therefore the probability of CHD, increases with increasing values of each of these variables, all other variables being kept constant. Sex and height have significant negative coefficients indicating that the probability of CHD is smaller with females and decreases with increasing height.

Furthermore, the logistic coefficients can be used to quantify the importance of each factor. The penultimate column of Table E11.5 contains the estimated relative risk (i.e. the odds ratio, see Chapter 15, p. 230) of getting CHD for each factor, after allowing for other prognostic factors. For example, the estimated relative risk of getting CHD for females compared with males is $\exp(b_i)$ = antilog $b_1 = 0.20$, i.e. the odds of getting CHD is 80% lower for females. The last column of Table E11.5 contains the approximate 95% confidence limits for each of the relative risks. In particular, the standard error of b_1, is estimated by $b_1/t_1 = 0.1742$, so that 95% confidence limits for the true logistic coefficient, β_1, are $-1.5883 \pm 2(0.1742) = -1.9367$ and -1.2399. Hence $\exp(\beta_1)$ has 95% confidence limits of $\exp(-1.9367)$ and $\exp(-1.2399) = 0.14$ and 0.29.

Chapter 12
Distribution-free Methods

Introduction

Hypothesis tests are often based on assumptions relating to the form of the data. Various procedures are available if these assumptions are not satisfied, e.g. (i) non-robust analyses; (ii) data transformations; and (iii) distribution-free analyses.

Non-robust analysis

Proceed with the test as prescribed, recognising that the validity of the resulting inferences may be in doubt; in particular, the significance level may be affected leading to a *non-robust* analysis. [A test is said to be *robust* against violations of its assumptions if the probabilities associated with the Type I error (rejecting H_0 when it is true) and the Type II error (not rejecting H_0 when it is false) are not appreciably affected by the violations.]

Data transformation

Procedure

Transform all of the original observations (x_i; $i = 1, 2, \ldots, n$) of the variable x to produce a new set of values ($y_i = f(x_i)$; $i = 1, 2, \ldots, n$), this transformed data set satisfying the needs of the analysis. Apply the appropriate statistical techniques to the transformed data.

Major applications

1. Equalisation of variances (e.g. two sample *t*-test, Chapter 8).
2. Linearisation of relationships.
3. Normalisation of distributions.

Common transformations

Logarithmic transformation

$$y = \log_e x = \ln x \text{ or } y = \log_{10} x.$$

Justification: (i) Normalises a positively skewed distribution [see Fig. 12.1(a) and (b)]. In particular, if a logarithmic transformation normalises the distribution of x, x has a *log-normal* distribution. (ii) Linearises a trend with a consistently increasing slope [see Fig. 12.1(c) and (d)]. The linearising effect of the transformation can be seen by either: (A) determining the logarithms of the values of x from logarithmic tables, and plotting these logarithmic values on an arithmetic scale [as in Fig. 12.1(d)]; or (B) using graph paper called *semi-logarithmic* paper on which the scale of x is specially calibrated, and plotting the arithmetic values of x on this scale. (iii) Equalises variances when the variance of x tends to increase markedly with x; more specifically, if the standard deviation of x varies directly as the mean [see Fig. 12.1(e) and (f)].

Square root transformation

$$y = \sqrt{x}.$$

Justification: Equalises variances when the variance of x tends to increase with x; more specifically, if the variance of x varies directly as the mean. In particular, the square root transformation is applied when x is a *count* of a rare event following the Poisson distribution.

Square transformation

$$y = x^2.$$

Justification: (i) Normalises a negatively skewed distribution. (ii) Linearises a trend with a consistently decreasing slope. (iii) Equalises variances if the variance of x tends to decrease with increasing x.

Transformations for a proportion, p

1. Angular: $y = \sin^{-1} \sqrt{p} = \arcsin \sqrt{p}$.
Justification: (i) Linearises a sigmoid curve [see Fig. 12.1(g) and (h)]. (ii) Equalises variances.

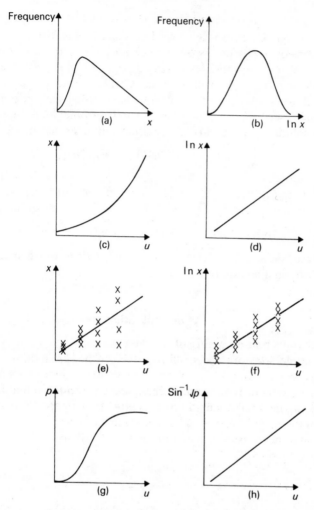

Fig. 12.1 Effects of common transformations.

2. Probit: $y = 5 + Z(1-p)$ where $Z(1-p)$ is the percentage point of the standard normal distribution beyond which lies $100(1-p)\%$ of the total probability.

Justification: Linearises a sigmoid curve.

Problem: If $p = 0$ or if $p = 1$ then y is indeterminable. An approximate solution is to obtain the percentage point, Z, from $p = 1/(2n)$ if $p = 0$, and from $p = 1 - 1/(2n)$ if $p = 1$.

3. Logit: $y = \log_e [p/(1-p)]$.

Justification: Linearises a sigmoid curve. The linearising effect of the transformation can be seen by either plotting the transformed values of p on arithmetically scaled paper or plotting the actual values of p on paper with one scale calibrated in a special way (called *probability* paper—analagous to semi-logarithmic paper).

Problem: If $p = 0$ or if $p = 1$ then y is indeterminable. An approximate solution is to modify the transformation so that it becomes

$$y = \log_e\{[p+1/(2n)]/[1-p+1/(2n)]\}$$

when $p = 0$ and $p = 1$.

Distribution-free (non-parametric) analysis

Replace the standard techniques by alternatives which make no distributional assumptions.

Major applications

1. Obvious non-normality of the data.
2. Sample sizes are too small to establish the distribution of the data.
3. Requirement is for rapid techniques, easy to learn and apply, involving minimal calculations, as is often so with distribution-free methods.
4. Data are measured by the ordinal (ranked) scale.

Remarks

1. Distribution-free methods are basically tests and are not adapted easily for purposes of estimation.
2. If all the assumptions of a parametric statistical test are met in the data, then non-parametric tests are wasteful of data. The degree of wastefulness may be expressed by the power-efficiency of the test, i.e. the ratio of sample sizes needed to provide a certain power in the two analogous tests.

Table 12.1 indicates some distribution-free alternatives to the parametric statistics discussed in previous chapters.

Table 12.1 Non-parametric alternatives to parametric statistics

Parametric	Non-parametric
Two sample t-test	Wilcoxon rank sum test
Paired t-test	Wilcoxon signed rank test
One-way analysis of variance	Kruskal–Wallis one-way analysis of variance*
Two-way analysis of variance	Friedman two-way analysis of variance*
Product moment correlation coefficient	Spearman's rank correlation coefficient

*The reader is referred to Siegel, S. (1956) *Non-parametric Statistics: for the Behavioral Sciences*. Tokyo: McGraw-Hill, pp. 184–193, and 166–172 for the Kruskal–Wallis and Friedman analysis of variance respectively.

Wilcoxon rank sum test

This is a distribution-free test comparing the distribution of observations in two populations, primarily with respect to location, using two *independent samples*.

Alternatives

Two other essentially equivalent distribution-free tests are: (i) Kendall's S test; and (ii) Mann–Whitney U test.

Procedure

Consider two populations, the set of observations $(x_1, x_2, \ldots, x_{N_1})$ from population X and the set of observations $(y_1, y_2, \ldots, y_{N_2})$ from population Y.

1. Define H_0: The distribution of x in population X is the same as that of y in population Y, primarily with respect to location. (*Note:* No specific reference is made to the means of the populations or to the forms of the distributions.)

2. Define H_1: The distributions of x in population X and y in population Y are different (no directional specification, say).

3. Select a random sample of n_1 observations $(x_1, x_2, \ldots, x_{n_1})$ from X and an *independent* random sample of n_2 observations $(y_1, y_2, \ldots, y_{n_2})$ from Y ($n_1 < n_2$, say).

4. Plot these sample values as shown in Fig. 8.1 (p. 72). The distributional forms of the sample values are unimportant. It may be useful to indicate the position of the median in each sample.

5. a. Rearrange the observations in both samples together so their values are of increasing magnitude, retaining the population identity of each observation. This is most easily achieved as follows: (i) order the observations in each sample *separately*, obtaining the ordered set $x_{(1)} \leq x_{(2)} \leq \ldots \leq x_{(n_1)}$ from X and the ordered set $y_{(1)} \leq y_{(2)} \leq \ldots \leq y_{(n_2)}$ from Y. The notation is that of Chapter 1. (ii) Order the observations in these two graded samples *together*, by drawing a horizontal line with the ordered observations from X (say) above the line and those from Y below the line, as shown in Fig. 12.2.

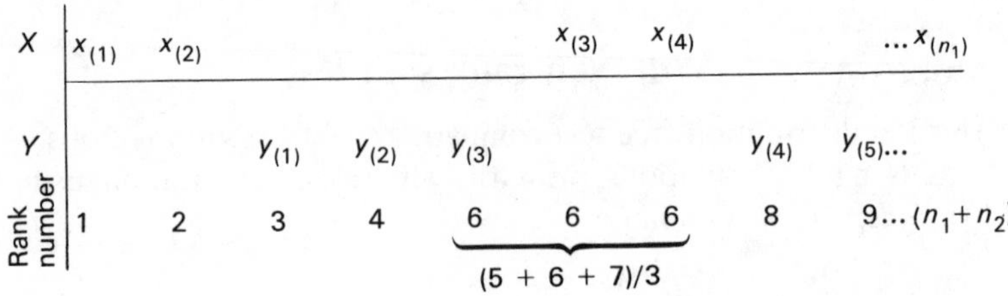

Fig. 12.2 Illustration of the ranking of two samples of observations for the Wilcoxon rank sum test. To illustrate the procedure for ties, it is assumed that $x_{(1)} = x_{(2)}$ and that $y_{(3)} = x_{(3)} = x_{(4)}$.

b. Assign successive *rank* numbers to the ordered observations in the two samples, where: (i) *tied* values within a sample receive successive rank numbers; (ii) *tied* values *between* the two samples each receive the arithmetic mean of the rank numbers they would have received had those values not been tied (see Fig. 12.2).
c. Consider the sum, T_{17}, of the rank numbers of the sample from population X (the smaller sample), and compute its value, T_{17C}, from the sample data. In the example of Fig. 12.2,

$$T_{17C} = 1+2+6+6+ \ldots +(n_1+n_2).$$

Determination of the sampling distribution of T_{17} depends on the sample sizes, n_1 and n_2.
i. $n_1+n_2 \leq 30$ ($2 \leq n_1 \leq 15$, $4 \leq n_2 \leq 28$).
The exact sampling distribution of T_{17} is determined. The reader is referred to Table A6 for significance limits, and should not proceed to steps 6 and 7.

ii. $n_1+n_2 > 30$.

The sampling distributions of T_{17} is approximately normal with mean $\mu_T = n_1(n_1+n_2+1)/2$ and variance $\sigma_T^2 = n_2\mu_T/6$*. The sampling distribution of the test statistic

$$T_{18} = (T_{17}-\mu_T)/\sigma_T$$

is approximately standard normal.

6. Compute the value, T_{18C}, of the test statistic from the sample data.

7. Determine the critical region from tables of the standard normal distribution (Table A1). For a two-tailed test at the $200\alpha\%$ level of significance, reject H_0 if $|T_{18C}|>Z(\alpha)$, $P < 2\alpha$. Do not reject H_0 otherwise, $P > 2\alpha$.

Wilcoxon signed rank test

This is a one sample distribution-free test for location. It is frequently used to compare two populations on the basis of two *related* samples, consisting of pairs of observations on individuals matched with respect to relevant extraneous variables.

Procedure

Consider two populations, the set of observations $(x_1, x_2, \ldots, x_N)$ from the population X and the set of observations $(y_1, y_2, \ldots, y_N)$ from population Y, with (x_i, y_i), $i = 1, 2, \ldots, N$, from a matched pair.

1. Define H_0: There is no difference in the distributions of x in X and y in Y for the members of a pair. The shape of the distribution need not be specified.

2. Define H_1: There is a difference in the distributions of x in X and y in Y for the members of a pair.

3. Select two random samples of observations, the set $(x_1, x_2, \ldots, x_{n_0})$ from population X and the set $(y_1, y_2, \ldots, y_{n_0})$ from population Y. The observations x_i and y_i $(i = 1, 2, \ldots, n_0)$

---

*If the proportion of ties is large, the variance formula should be modified to

$$\frac{n_1n_2}{12n(n-1)} \left[n^3-n-\sum_t (t^3-t) \right]$$

where the summation is taken over all groups of tied observations, t being the number of observations in a particular group, and $n = n_1+n_2$.

are a pair of observations on two matched individuals or on one individual on two occasions.

4. Plot these sample values, most easily using the same scale of measurement for each sample, as shown in Fig. 8.3 (p. 77). Retain the basic information of the pairings by joining the two observations in each pair by a straight line.

5. a. For each matched pair, determine the signed *difference* between its sample values. For the ith pair ($i = 1, 2, \ldots, n_0$), this difference is $d_i = x_i - y_i$. Zero differences are ignored so henceforth consideration is given only to the n (say) non-zero differences ($n \leqslant n_0$).

b. Rearrange the absolute (without regard to sign) values of the differences, ($|d_1|, |d_2|, \ldots, |d_n|$), in increasing order of magnitude, producing the set $|d|_{(1)} \leqslant |d|_{(2)} \leqslant \ldots \leqslant |d|_{(n)}$. Retain the information of the sign of each difference, most easily by drawing a horizontal line with positive (say) differences above it and negative differences below it (see Fig. 12.3).

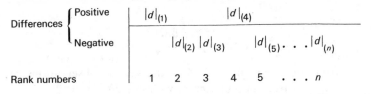

Fig. 12.3 Illustration of ranking of a sample of absolute differences for the Wilcoxon signed rank test.

c. Assign successive *rank numbers* to the ordered absolute differences. The procedure adopted for tied values corresponds to that described for the Wilcoxon rank sum test (see Fig. 12.3).

d. Consider the sum, T_{19}, of the rank numbers of the like-signed differences, i.e. the sum of the rank numbers of the positive differences above the line or the sum of the rank numbers of the negative differences below the line, whichever is smaller, and compute its value, T_{19C}, from the sample data. Determination of the sampling distribution of T_{19} depends on n, the number of non-zero differences in the sample.

i. $n \leqslant 25$:

The exact sampling distribution of T_{19} is determined. The reader is referred to Table A7 for significance limits, and should not proceed to steps 6 and 7.

ii. $n > 25$:

The sampling distribution of T_{19} is approximately normal with mean $n(n+1)/4$ and variance $n(n+1)(2n+1)/24$*. Thus the sampling distribution of the test statistic

$$T_{20} = [T_{19}-n(n+1)/4]/\sqrt{n(n+1)(2n+1)/24}$$

is approximately standard normal.

6. Compute the value, T_{20C}. of the test statistic from the sample data.

7. Determine the critical region from the tables of the standard normal distribution (Table A1). For a two-tailed test at the $200\alpha\%$ level of significance, reject H_0 if $|T_{20C}| > Z(\alpha)$, $P < 2\alpha$. Do not reject H_0 otherwise, $P > 2\alpha$.

Spearman's rank correlation coefficient

Although two distribution-free correlation coefficients, Kendall's tau (τ) and Spearman's rho (ρ_s), are in common usage, only the latter is discussed. It gives a measure of the association between two variables, x and y.

Applications

The procedure is used in one or more of the following cases: (i) the n pairs of sample observations $[(x_1, y_1), (x_2, y_2), \ldots, (x_n, y_n)]$ do *not* come from a bivariate *normal* distribution; (ii) at least one of the variables x and y is measured on an ordinal (ranked) scale; (iii) a measure is required which does not rely on the concept of closeness to linear regression.

Definition

Spearman's rank correlation coefficient, ρ_s, is estimated in a random sample of n pairs of observations $[(x_1, y_1), (x_2, y_2) \ldots, (x_n, y_n)]$ by

$$r_s = 1 - \frac{6\sum d_i^2}{n^3-n}$$

*If the proportion of ties is large, the variance formula should be reduced by $(t^3-t)/48$ for each group of t tied ranks.

where d_i = difference between the rank number of x_i in the set $(x_1, x_2, \ldots, x_n)$ and the rank number of y_i in the set $(y_1, y_2, \ldots, y_n)$ for the ith individual.

Method

1. Assign the appropriate rank numbers $1, 2, \ldots, n$ to each of the values $x_1, x_2, \ldots, x_n$.
2. Assign the appropriate rank numbers $1, 2, \ldots, n$ to each of the values $y_1, y_2, \ldots, y_n$.
3. List the n individuals, specifying for the ith individual ($i = 1, 2, \ldots, n$) the rank number of x_i and the rank number of y_i.
4. Determine the difference d_i for the ith individual ($i = 1, 2, \ldots, n$) by subtracting the rank number of y_i from the rank number of x_i.
5. Calculate r_s using the formula above.

Ties

When the value of a variable is the same in two or more individuals, each individual is assigned the average of the rank numbers which would have been assigned had no ties occurred. If the proportion of ties is large, the formula for r_s should be modified. The reader is referred to Seigel, S. (1956), p. 207.

Properties of r_s

1. $-1 \leqslant r_s \leqslant +1$.
2. r_s is the ordinary sample product moment correlation coefficient between the rank numbers of x and y.

Hypothesis test of ρ_s

1. Define H_0: $\rho_s = 0$. (There is no association between x and y).
2. Define H_1: $\rho_s \neq 0$. (There is an association between x and y, direction unspecified.)
3. Select a random sample of n pairs of observations $[(x_1, y_1), (x_2, y_2), \ldots, (x_n, y_n)]$ from the population.
4. Draw a scatter diagram of the sample observations and observe the form of the relationship, if any, between the variables.
5. Consider the sample Spearman's rank correlation coefficient,

r_s. Determination of the sampling distribution of r_s depends on the sample size, n.

a. *Small n:*

The exact sampling distribution of r_s is determined. The reader is referred to pp. 66–67 of *Documenta Geigy Scientific Tables* (1970) for significance limits for $5 \leqslant n \leqslant 199$ (these limits are exact only for $1 \leqslant n \leqslant 10$), and need not proceed to steps **6** and **7**.

b. *Large n:*

As an alternative to using the table specified above giving approximate limits for large n, consider the test statistic

$$T_{21} = r_s \sqrt{\frac{n-2}{1-r_s^2}}$$

whose sampling distribution is t on $n-2$ degrees of freedom, for large enough n. The reader is referred to Kendall, M. G. (1955), for the justification of T_{21}.

6. Compute the value, T_{21C}, of the test statistic from the sample data.

7. Determine the critical region from tables of the t-distribution (Table A3). For a two-tailed test at the $200\alpha\%$ level of significance, reject H_0 if $|T_{21C}| > t_{n-2}(\alpha)$, $P < 2\alpha$. Do not reject H_0 otherwise, $P > 2\alpha$.

Examples

Wilcoxon rank sum test

1. H_0: The distribution of the synthesis of alkaline phosphatase is the same in normal subjects and non-responsive coeliac patients.

2. H_1: The distributions are different.

3. A random sample of six normal subjects is selected as well as an independent random sample of seven non-responsive coeliac patients. The synthesis of alkaline phosphatase is measured in each subject and the results are presented in Table E12.1.

Table E12.1 Synthesis of alkaline phosphate (mU/µg DNA) in two groups of individuals

Normals	0.46	0.46	0.56	0.42	0.51	0.77	
Coeliacs	1.60	0.77	0.80	1.62	1.32	1.10	0.75

Source: P. E. Jones (personal communication).

4. The data are presented in Fig. E12.1. The distribution of the observations in each sample is skewed. In view of this and the fact that each observation is in reality a ratio of two random variables (the sampling distribution of a ratio is not easy to determine), it is advisable to consider a non-parametric test.

Normals	0.42	0.46	0.46	0.51	0.56		0.77						
Coeliacs							0.75		0.77	0.80	1.10	1.32	1.60	1.62
Rank no.	1	2	3	4	5		6	7.5	7.5	9	10	11	12	13

Fig. E12.1 Ordered values of synthesis of alkaline phosphatase (mU/μg DNA) in normal subjects and non-responsive coeliac patients.

5. a. (i) The ordered observations (each sample separately) are: *Normals:* 0.42, 0.46, 0.46, 0.51, 0.56, 0.77 [$n_1 = 6$, median $= (0.46+0.51)/2 = 0.485$]. *Coeliacs:* 0.75, 0.77, 0.80, 1.10, 1.32, 1.60, 1.62 ($n_2 = 7$, median $= 1.10$). (ii) The ordered observations (the two samples together) are shown in Fig. E12.1.
b. Successive rank numbers are assigned to the ordered observations, as shown in Fig. E12.1.
c. Consider the sum, T_{17}, of the rank numbers of the smaller sample (normals).
6. Its value computed from the sample data is

$$T_{17C} = 1+2+3+4+5+7.5 = 22.5.$$

7. Referring to Table A6, the tabulated critical value of T_{17} when $n_1 = 6$, $n_2 = 7$ is 23 (when $2\alpha = 0.01$). Thus since $T_{17C} < 23$, significance is achieved at the 1% level and H_0 is rejected, $P < 0.01$.

Wilcoxon signed rank test

It is of interest to investigate the ability of a new fluoride containing toothpaste to slow down the development of tooth decay in children as measured by the DMFS increment over a period of 3 years.

1. H_0: There is no difference in the ability of the new fluoride denifrice and a non-fluoride denifrice to slow down the tooth decay in children.
2. H_1: There is a difference.

3. A random sample of 13 children is selected and each child in the sample matched with another child of the same social class, age, sex, with an equal oral hygiene score who claims to brush his (her) teeth with equal frequency. One child of the matched pair is selected at random and provided with the fluoride toothpaste; the other member of the pair is given a similar non-fluoride toothpaste. After a period of 3 years, during which the children are checked, their teeth are again examined and the number of tooth surfaces which have decayed since the start of the trial (DMFS increment) counted. The results are presented in Table E12.2. The distribution of the increments in those children receiving the non-fluoride toothpaste is skewed. In view of this and the fact that the increments are counts (Poisson distribution), it is advisable to consider a non-parametric test.

Table E12.2 DMFS increments in pairs of children receiving two types of toothpaste

Pair	1	2	3	4	5	6	7	8	9	10	11	12	13
Non-fluoride	9	10	4	19	13	12	8	0	13	6	12	5	7
Fluoride	6	7	3	19	4	12	2	0	16	7	5	0	7
Difference	3	3	1	0	9	0	6	0	−3	−1	7	5	0

Source: Hypothetical data.
Note: median DMFS increment = 1.

4. The sample values are presented in Fig. E12.2.
5. a. For each pair of children, the signed difference in the increments between the members of a pair receiving the non-fluoride and fluoride toothpastes is determined, as shown in Table E12.2.

Differences	Positive	1		3	3		5	6	7	9
	Negative		1			3				
Rank numbers		1.5	1.5	4	4	4	6	7	8	9
		(1+2)/2		(3+4+5)/3						

Fig. E12.2 Ordered absolute differences in DMFS increments between two toothpastes.

b. The absolute values of these differences (ignoring zero differences) are arranged in order of magnitude, as shown in Fig. E12.2.

c. Successive rank numbers are assigned to these absolute differences, as shown in Fig. E12.2.

d. Consider the sum, T_{19}, of the rank numbers of the like-signed differences.

6. Its value computed from the sample data is

$$T_{19C} = 1.5 + 4 = 5.5.$$

7. Referring to Table A7, the tabulated critical values of T_{19} when $n = 9$ are 6 (when $2\alpha = 0.05$) and 2 (when $2\alpha = 0.01$). Since $T_{19C} < 6$ but $T_{19C} > 2$, significance is achieved at the 5% level and H_0 is rejected, $0.01 < P < 0.05$.

Remark

An alternative method of testing H_0 is by the *sign test*. If there is no difference between the fluoride and non-fluoride toothpastes in slowing down the development of tooth decay in children (as measured by the DMFS increment), then positive and negative differences in DMFS increments are equally likely. If π is the true proportion of positive differences in DMFS increments between the fluoride and non-fluoride toothpastes in the population, then an equivalent expression of H_0 is $H_0: \pi = 1/2$. The test is thus one of a proportion (Chapter 7). The procedure is:

1. $H_0: \pi = 1/2 = 0.5$.

2. $H_1: \pi \neq 1/2$.

3. The DMFS increments in a random sample of 13 matched pairs of children are given in Table E12.2. There are nine non-zero differences in the increments between the fluoride and non-fluoride toothpastes; seven of these are positive.

4. No visual presentation.

5. Consider

$$T_3 = [|p - \pi_0| - 1/(2n)]/\sqrt{\pi_0(1 - \pi_0)/n}$$

where $p = 7/9 = 0.78$, the sample estimate of π; $\pi_0 = 0.5$; $n = 9$.

6.
$$T_{3C} = [|0.78-0.5|-1/(18)]/\sqrt{(0.5)(0.5)/9}$$
$$= 1.35.$$

7. From tables of the standard normal distribution (Table A1), $Z(0.025) = 1.96$. Hence $|T_{3C}| < Z(0.025)$ since $1.35 < 1.96$. Thus do not reject H_0, $P > 0.05$ [*note:* the sign test loses information by ignoring the magnitude of the differences—it considers only the sign of each difference. This accounts for the fact that H_0 is not rejected ($P > 0.05$) when the sign test is performed on the given data set, whilst the Wilcoxon signed rank test (using more information) rejects H_0 ($0.01 < P < 0.05$) on the basis of the same data set].

Spearman's rank correlation coefficient

Consider the data of Table E11.1. Arranged in ascending order of magnitude the ages (years) of the 10 patients are:

24 26 34 36 37 39 44 45 47 53.

The 6 hour postoperative Pa_{O_2} measurements (mm Hg) arranged in ascending order of magnitude are:

74 76 78 82 86 87 91 94 95 99.

The appropriate rank numbers between 1 and 10 are assigned to the ages and the Pa_{O_2} measurements of the 10 patients, as shown in Table E12.3. The difference, and its square, between the rank numbers for each patient are also shown in the table.

Table E12.3 Rank numbers of the age and 6 hour postoperative Pa_{O_2} measurements of 10 patients receiving 50% nitrous oxide with oxygen during varicose vein operations

Patient (i)	1	2	3	4	5	6	7	8	9	10	Total
Rank of age	9	2	3	4	1	8	6	5	7	10	
Rank of Pa_{O_2}	1	7	3	10	8	2	9	4	5	6	
Difference in ranks (d_i)	8	−5	0	−6	−7	6	−3	1	2	4	
d_i^2	64	25	0	36	49	36	9	1	4	16	240

Source: Table E11.1.

Then

$$r_s = 1 - \frac{6 \sum d_i^2}{n^3 - n}$$

$$= 1 - \frac{6(240)}{1000 - 10}$$

$$= -0.45.$$

Note: By coincidence, this corresponds exactly to the sample product moment correlation coefficient calculated in the Examples to Chapter 11.

Hypothesis test of ρ_s

1. H_0: $\rho_s = 0$.
2. H_1: $\rho_s \neq 0$.
3. A random sample of 10 patients who undergo varicose vein operations receiving 50% nitrous oxide with oxygen is selected. The ages and 6 hour postoperative measurements of Pao_2 of these patients are shown in Table E11.1.
4. Figure E.11.1 is a scatter diagram of the sample observations.
5. Spearman's rank correlation coefficient is estimated in the sample as -0.45 (see above). Since n is small ($n = 10$), reference is made to the significance limits given on pp. 66–67 of *Documenta Geigy Scientific Tables* (1970). From the sample, $\sum d_i^2 = 240$ (see Table E12.3) which lies within the upper (272) and lower (58) 5% significance limits given in *Documenta Geigy*. Hence do not reject H_0 that Spearman's rank correlation coefficient is zero, $P > 0.05$ (c.f. the test of H_0: $\rho = 0$, p. 163).

Chapter 13
Clinical Trials

Clinical trials

Although the fundamental rules for conducting clinical trials on a scientific basis were only established in the early 1950s (in great part due to the work of Sir Austin Bradford-Hill), the growth of methodology in this area since then has been enormous. Thus no attempt is made here to give a detailed account of the present state of statistical knowledge about clinical trials, with their related ethical and organisational difficulties. Instead, the principles and problems are outlined. The reader is referred to Pocock, S. J. (1984) for a full discussion.

Definition

Clinical trials are planned experiments comparing the efficacy of different medical treatments when they are administered to patients. They are often called *controlled* clinical trials in that they invariably utilise a control group of patients receiving a standard treatment, if available, or no active treatment as a comparative gauge to elucidate the effect of a new treatment. (An *uncontrolled* trial generally provides a distorted view of therapy and, in particular, is more likely to lead to an enthusiastic recommendation of the new treatment than a properly controlled trial.) Furthermore, as *randomisation* is usually adopted as a mechanism for overcoming bias (see pp. 191–195), the majority of trials are *randomised controlled clinical trials*.

Uses

Clinical trials may involve:

1. Drug comparisons (i) against each other; (ii) against a standard treatment; (iii) against a dummy treatment; and (iv) in the absence of effective treatment.

187

2. Surgery.
3. Irradiation.
4. Cross comparisons of different categories; e.g. surgery *vs* drug.
5. Vaccines.
6. Paramedical treatments, e.g. forms of medical care or health education.

Phases of investigation

A clinical trial is generally preceded by preliminary investigations of the treatment on animals and healthy volunteers, only then progressing to the following clinical phases:

1. *Initial trial*—on a few patients:
   a. To establish safety.
   b. To determine possible non-toxic schedules.
   c. To assess possible therapeutic effects (essentially a screening procedure).
2. *Confirmatory trial*—a full scale comparative trial on more patients.
3. *Familiarisation trial*—an extension of the confirmatory trial of a more pragmatic nature involving: (i) a greater exposure of patients; (ii) more clinicians, often non-specialists (e.g. general practitioners).

Discussion in this chapter is restricted to the confirmatory trial.

Ethical problems

Ethical problems arise in various forms in clinical trials, the most prominent being, perhaps, whether it is proper to withold from any patient a treatment from which he might derive benefit. Other areas leading to ethical difficulties include (i) the process of randomisation of patients to the various treatments; (ii) the administration of a placebo or dummy treatment; (iii) the acquisition of truly 'informed' patient consent to be included in the trial and (iv) the propriety of a double-blind trial in which the clinician is ignorant of the treatment that he is administering to a particular patient.

Publications

The major treatises on medical ethics are: (i) Code of the World

Medical Association (1960, revised 1975)*, i.e. the Nuremberg Rules or Declaration of Helsinki; (ii) Directives of the Medical Research Council (1963)*; (iii) Report by the Royal College of Physicians (1967); (iv) Report by the World Health Organization Scientific Group (1968); and (v) *The Handbook of Medical Ethics* by the British Medical Association (1980).

Solution to the ethical dilemma

The clinical trial is justified only when the clinician involved maintains an *'agnostic'* attitude as to the benefits of the participatory treatments, all of which are known, as far as possible, not to be detrimental to the patient. It is the clinician's duty to administer the best known treatment to each patient. A lack of knowledge of the 'best' remedy provides a framework from which the clinical trial evolves.

In reality, the clinician adopts an attitude of 'collective' (as distinct from 'individual') ethics, permitting the accumulation of reliable data for the benefit of future patients, provided that there is no clear indication that the interests of his present patients are damaged.

A general criterion proposed for the propriety of a trial is that it is not ethical unless the clinician would allow himself or a near relative to be included in it.

Safeguards

It is impossible to define absolute criteria for a code of practice. A compromise solution is to provide safeguards to the patients and clinicians, e.g. (i) employ ethical committees; (ii) retain the right to withdraw patients from the trial; (iii) obtain the patient's informed consent to be included in the trial. If he is legally incompetent, the consent of the legal guardian should be procured; (iv) avoid inducements to attract volunteers.

Role of the statistician

1. *Bias*: He provides safeguards against bias by devising experiments free from systematic errors of allocation and assessment.

*Partly printed in Pocock, S. J. (1983) *Clinical Trials. A Practical Approach.* Chichester; Wily, pp. 100–102.

2. *Critical approach*: He is able to look critically at the pertinence of the intended measurements to the objectives of the trial.

3. *Analysis*: He uses his technical skills to ensure the appropriate analysis is performed.

4. *Efficiency*: He is able to increase the efficiency of the trial by utilising the minimal number of patients to provide the relevant information. The choice of *sample size* is dependent on a number of factors. In the simple situation in which two treatments are compared, these factors are usually:

    a. A specification of the difference in the responses to the two treatments, δ, which is deemed important and should not be overlooked.

    b. A specification of the maximum allowable probability associated with the Type I error, α (often 0.05).

    c. A specification of the maximum allowable probability associated with the Type II error, β (often 0.10). An equivalent specification is of the power of the test at δ, $(1-\beta)$, representing the probability of detecting a specified difference, δ, in response to the two treatments. Clearly, a powerful study (one with a high probability of detecting a specified important treatment difference) is desirable. For a prescribed Type I error, the power of the test increases when the sample size increases.

    d. A knowledge of the variation in the data, assimilated possibly from earlier trials or as a result of a *pilot* trial. (A pilot investigation is an investigation usually on a small scale, carried out prior to the main investigation, primarily to gain information to improve the efficiency of the main investigation.)

The reader is referred to Armitage, P. (1987), pp. 179–185, for a full explanation and formulae.

Sometimes sufficient numbers of patients for a viable trial cannot be obtained from a single source and a *multi-centre* trial may be warranted. The main advantage of a multi-centre trial is that patient accrual is quicker so that more reliable conclusions of more general applicability can be reached at a faster rate. However, this advantage must be balanced by the complexities of planning, administration and data processing, the expense and difficulties of obtaining uniformity. The reader is referred to Pocock, S. J. (1984), pp. 134–138, for a full discussion.

Trial design

A clinical trial is an experiment and thus the design of the trial must take account of the relevant principles of experimental design. The most important of these are: (i) removal of systematic errors of allocation; (ii) elimination of systematic errors of assessment; and (iii) replication in the study of random variation.

Removal of systematic errors of allocation

When testing for differences in response between the treatment groups, it is important to ensure that the groups are similar in all respects (e.g. weight, age) other than the treatments they receive. This may be achieved by the methods outlined below.

Matching

The patients are matched in the treatment groups so that the groups are alike with respect to any variable thought to influence response.

Disadvantage: It may not be possible to determine, in advance, those variables which influence response and introduce bias.

Randomisation

Each patient is randomly (by chance methods) allocated to one of the treatment groups.

ADVANTAGES OF RANDOMISATION

1. Bias is eliminated from the assignment of patients to treatments.
2. Treatment groups tend to be balanced in covariates (prognostic factors) whether or not these variables are known.
3. Blind allocation (see p. 196) is facilitated by randomisation.
4. The validity of statistical tests of significance that are used to compare the treatments is guaranteed.

RANDOMISATION *VS* HISTORICAL CONTROLS

When information is available about the efficacy of a standard treatment through historical data, then it can be argued that it is

preferable to use these *historical controls* in a trial rather than the
concurrent controls obtained by randomising the patients to the
new and standard treatment groups.

The use of historical controls has the *advantages* that all patients
in the trial receive the new treatment which the investigators expect
to be superior, there is a substantial saving in the number of patients
required and therefore, generally, in the length of the study. Some
of the arguments against randomisation forwarded by the pro-
tagonists of historical controls are listed and countered in Table
13.1.

Table 13.1 Arguments against randomisation with counterarguments

Arguments against randomisation	Counterarguments
It is unethical to allow a random event determine a patient's treatment	If the physician's attitude to the relative merits of the participatory treatments is 'agnostic' (see p. 189) then the process of randomisation does not exacerbate the ethical difficulties. A proper ethical stance is to propose a randomised controlled trial to obtain a credible and hopefully definitive answer to the question of treatment superiority
A comparative trial which shows major differences between the effects of new and standard treatments is unethical because half the patients will have received the inferior treatment	The differences between the effects of treatments only emerge *after* the trial has been conducted
When the benefit to be derived from the new treatment is believed to be exceptionally great then it is not necessary, and probably unethical, to allocate some patients to the standard (or no) treatment group	The new treatment is only known to be superior, with any degree of certainty, *after* the trial has been conducted
If the disease under investigation is rare, then it is difficult to accumulate enough patients for a randomised controlled study in which half the patients receive the new treatment	The difficulty can be overcome by collaborative effort or multi-centre trials

The *problem* with trials using historical controls (whether
obtained from a previous trial or a collection of historical data

from within the same organisation, or, most particularly, from the literature) is that they provide limited protection against the biases introduced by changes in the nature of the patient population, in exposure to pathological agents and in supportive care and diagnostic criteria. The net effect of these biases is that studies with historical controls tend to exaggerate the value of a new treatment. Post hoc adjustment procedures that attempt to correct for possible bias due to an imbalance in prognostic factors are available but the validity of these techniques depends on the correctness of the assumed mathematical model.

It is therefore generally, but not universally, agreed that clinical trials should use randomised controls, although not necessarily in the conventional manner with equally sized treatment groups. In particular, the following two compromise situations have been suggested:

1. Unequal randomisation in which more than half the random assignments are to the new treatment. The randomisation in a 2:1 or 3:2 ratio for new:standard treatment is quite acceptable. Any ratio equal to, or more extreme than, 3:1 results in a considerable loss of power and is probably undesirable.

2. Both randomised controls and historical controls are utilised in the same trial instead of relying exclusively on one or the other; see Pocock, S. J. (1976), for details.

METHODS OF RANDOMISATION

Random allocation may be executed using:

Mechanical methods

Two examples are (i) toss a coin (for two treatments, 'Heads' designates one treatment and 'Tails', the other); (ii) roll a dice (for six treatments, each face designates a different treatment).

Disadvantages: (i) cumbersome and time-consuming; (ii) not repeatable, cannot be subsequently checked.

Table of random numbers (Table A8)

The digits 0–9 are arranged in random order. By progressing up or down one or more adjacent columns (or along one or more adjacent rows) of digits, it is possible to allocate the patients randomly to the treatments. The following two examples illustrate the method.

1. *Trial size, n, known.*

    a. Assign the numbers $1-n$ to each of the patients.

    b. Record the numbers $1-n$ as they occur in the sequence of digits in the table of random numbers to obtain a random permutation (variation in the order) of n. Ignore repetitions and numbers greater than n in the sequence.

    c. To allocate randomly the n patients to k treatments groups, divide the random permutation of n from left to right into groups of the appropriate size. The numbers contained in each group correspond to those patients who receive a specified treatment. For example, if $n = 10$ and $k = 2$ (the two groups being of equal size) and the random permutation is 5 4 10 2 1 6 8 7 9 3, then the first five numbers in the random permutation of 10 (i.e. 5 4 10 2 1) correspond to those patients who receive one treatment, whilst the second five numbers in the random permutation of 10 (i.e. the remaining numbers 6 8 7 9 3) correspond to those patients who receive the other treatment.

2. *Trial size, n, unknown*

    a. Unrestricted randomisation.

        (i) Enter the patients serially.

        (ii) To each patient in turn allot the number obtained by following a random sequence of digits in the random number table.

        (iii) Allocate each patient to the treatment group determined by the interpretation of his number. This interpretation depends essentially on the number of treatment groups. For example, for equal probability allocation of:

        (A) two treatments, T_1, T_2: Allocate the patient to T_1 if his number is odd. Allocate the patient to T_2 if his number is even.

        (B) three treatments, T_1, T_2, T_3: Allocate the patient to T_1 if his number is 1, 2 or 3. Allocate the patient to T_2 if his number is 4, 5 or 6. Allocate the patient to T_3 if his number is 7, 8 or 9. Ignore 0.

b. Restricted randomisation.

It is generally advantageous to have equal numbers of patients in all of the treatment groups. If the trial size, n, is initially unknown, this may be achieved by ensuring that the numbers allocated to the different treatments are equal at various stages.

(i) Decide on a number b (e.g. 4, 10, 20) which determines that the numbers in all treatment groups be balanced after every multiple of b.

(ii) Enter the patients serially and separate them into groups of size b.

(iii) To every group of b patients, apply the technique described for random allocation when the trial size is known. In this instance, the 'trial size' is b instead of n (e.g. if $b = 10$ and the number of treatments $k = 2$, then five patients are randomly allocated to one treatment and the remaining five are allocated to the other treatment, balance being achieved after every 10, 20, 30, . . . patients). The numbers in the treatment groups are exactly balanced after every b patients, and are approximately balanced after the total intake of n patients if b is not a multiple of n.

Stratification and randomisation

The numbers entering the study may be small in which case randomisation may not fully remove the bias arising from the allocation of patients to treatments; or it may be necessary to study certain *strata* (divisions of the population: e.g. the two strata, male and female, defining the sex categories) separately. In such cases it may be worthwhile to stratify the patients as they enter the study and then randomly allocate the patients to the treatment groups within each stratum.

Within-patient studies

The composition of different treatment groups can be made identical by designing the trial so that each patient receives all treatments. The treatment comparisons are then made within-patients rather than between-patients, generally achieving a greater precision. Such *cross-over* trials are most naturally made in studies of short-term relief of chronic diseases. The order in which the patients receive the treatments is determined randomly to remove any order-related bias. Care should be taken to ensure there is no carry-over effect from one treatment period to the next. The reader is referred to Hills, M. and Armitage, P. (1979) for details.

Elimination of systematic errors of assessment

Biases may arise because of the often subjective nature of the assessment of response to treatment and the preconceived notions of the patient and/or clinician. Such biases may be overcome using one or more of the following techniques.

Single-blind

The patient is unaware of which treatment he is receiving. A single-blind trial removes assessment bias when the patient, rather than the clinician, assesses the response to treatment. The treatments should appear alike in all respects to avoid detection at the stage of administration.

Double-blind

Neither the clinician assessing response nor the patient is aware of which treatment the patient is receiving. The treatments should be indistinguishable at the stage of administration.

Disadvantages: (i) A potential loss of faith in the clinician by the patient because the clinician is 'without knowledge'; (ii) possible organisational difficulties.

Placebo

This is a pharmacologically inert dummy, identical in appearance to the treatment(s), which dissociates the specific pharmacological effect of the treatment(s) from the suggestive element imposed by the receipt of treatment.

Uses: (i) It is unethical to use a placebo when a known effective treatment exists; (ii) the placebo may be used as a *double-dummy* when the treatments cannot be presented in identical forms; e.g. if the effect of a cream is to be compared with that of a tablet, a placebo cream and a placebo tablet are prepared and the comparison (cream+placebo tablet) *vs* (tablet+placebo cream) is made.

Replication in the study of random variation

Inherent in the study of response to treatment is the presence of random variation which cannot be attributed to any specific factor (e.g. treatments, patients, times) but is usually regarded as a consequence of methodological errors and the effects of miscellaneous fluctuating factors. This random variation may be compared with the variation resulting from the differences in the levels of each of the factors under study, as a means of determining whether those differences are significant. Generally, not all the factors in the study are of intrinsic interest but by separating out the variation of the components, it is possible to establish the magnitude of the differences in the levels of the factors that are of interest. Thus, it is important to design the trial so that the variation due to any relevant factors can be quantified. In addition, *replication* of the number of experimental units and of the number of repeat observations per experimental unit is a means of increasing precision.

The reader is referred to Cox, D. R. (1958) for a full discussion.

Sequential analysis

The patients are drawn one by one or in groups in order, and the results at any stage decide whether sampling is to continue; i.e. there are multiple assessments of results through time. The trial size is not fixed in advance but depends on the actual results.

The sampling terminates according to predetermined *stopping-rules* which are decided, in general, by specifying the same quantities needed for the determination of sample size in a non-sequential trial; e.g. the probabilities associated with the Type I and Type II errors, the differences in response to treatment considered important and the variation in the data. From this information, a *chart* is constructed in which the stopping rules are presented pictorially as boundary lines. The results are plotted on the chart as they become available, the decision being taken to *carry on sampling* if the most recent result lies within the boundaries and to *stop* in favour of one or other of the treatments (generally, a sequential trial compares only two treatments) if that result crosses a boundary, each boundary representing a preference for a different treatment. In addition, a middle boundary is generally included in the chart as a means of avoiding the possibility of exceptionally large sample sizes. If the most recent result crosses this closure boundary then the decision is taken to stop sampling and the conclusion drawn that there is no significant difference between the treatments.

An *example* of a sequential chart to compare two treatments, A and B, is given in Fig. 13.1. The horizontal scale measures the number of preferences recorded at any stage; the vertical scale measures the 'excess preferences', i.e. the difference between the number of preferences in favour of treatment A and the number of preferences in favour of treatment B.

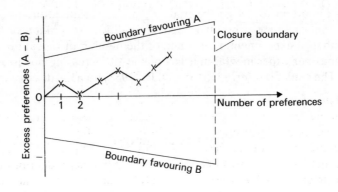

Fig. 13.1 Sequential chart for a series of preferences, with a sample of results.

Suitable circumstances of use

1. Patients are started on treatment serially in time.

2. Assessments of response to treatments become available in sequential order.

3. The time between administration of and response to treatment is short in comparison to the rate of entry of patients to the trial; e.g. in acute conditions or for rapid relief of chronic conditions.

4. There is a single response of primary importance which can be used to assess the treatments. The decision whether to stop or not at any stage is based on this response so that any other forms of response will probably be compared with less precision.

Advantages of sequential trials

Economy

On the average, the sample size in a sequential trial is less than that of the analogous fixed sample size trial.

Ethics

Sequential trials allow continuous scrutiny of results and avoid extensive experimentation when treatment differences are large, both facets being ethically advantageous.

The reader is referred to Armitage, P. (1975) for a full discussion.

Group sequential trial designs (repeated significance tests)

Many clinical trials stipulate that, in order to fulfil ethical obligations, random allocation should cease if it becomes reasonably apparent that one treatment is superior to the other(s). The sequential methods outlined above meet this ethical requirement and are concerned with *continuous* monitoring of the accumulating data. In practice, such methods are rarely feasible and the *analysis of interim results at periodic intervals* (i.e., repeated significance tests) is an alternative and often preferred procedure which falls between single-sample and strictly sequential methods. However, if these interim analyses are performed in a casual way then there will be a higher probability of finding a significant difference between the treatments purely by chance (in the absence of a real treatment difference) than if the tests were performed once, at the final stage of the trial (see corresponding argument against performing multiple *t*-tests, p. 78). To overcome this difficulty, the methods for interim analyses are formalised and well defined in particular instances. (Theoretical results are generally confined to two treatments each with a normal response variable with known variance, σ^2, and to two-sided significance tests, although simulation studies have shown they adapt to other types of response data.) See Pocock, S. J. (1977) and Pocock, S. J. (1982) for full discussions.

Outline of method

The technique depends on the distinction between:

1. The *nominal* significance level, α'—the significance level used for each repeated test. This is generally held constant throughout a trial and is more stringent than

2. the *overall* significance level, α—the probability associated with the risk of a false positive finding. It is generally set to some desired level, such as 0.05, and the nominal significance level determined accordingly.

Table 13.2 (extracted from Pocock, S. J. 1983) relates the nominal and overall significance levels for different values of N, the maximum number of tests.

Table 13.2 Nominal significance levels*, α', for repeated two-sided significance testing with overall significance levels $\alpha = 0.05$ and $\alpha = 0.01$ and various values of N, the maximum number of tests

N	$\alpha = 0.05$	$\alpha = 0.01$
2	0.029	0.0056
3	0.022	0.0041
4	0.018	0.0033
5	0.016	0.0028

*These nominal levels are exactly true for a normally distributed response with known variance, but are also a good approximation for many other types of data.

In essence, the *procedure* is to decide, at the planning stage of the trial, how many interim analyses are to be performed and then to proceed with the specified number of significance tests, using the relevant nominal significance level on equally sized patient groups at all intermediate stages. For example, with at most five analyses and overall Type I error $= 0.05$, $P < 0.016$ is adopted as a shopping rule for a treatment difference for each analysis.

Trial size

Clearly, the technique relies on an initial specification of the number of patients required for each interim analysis. As with a 'one-look' fixed sample size trial, the optimal trial size can be determined using power considerations (see p. 190).

It can be shown that although a group sequential trial design requires more patients than a 'one-look' fixed sample size trial if the null hypothesis of no treatment difference is true (in which circumstances, fortunately, there is no ethical dilemma), the group sequential design has the important *advantage* that it enables early termination (so that the average number of patients is less) if the null hypothesis is false and a treatment difference exists.

Optimal number of interim analyses

It can be shown that there is little statistical advantage in undertaking more than *five* interim analyses during the course of the trial, unless extremely large treatment differences are anticipated. Furthermore, a trial with just *two* analyses (one half way through, and one at the end) has considerable advantage over a 'one-look' fixed sample size trial in reducing the average number of patients exposed to an inferior treatment.

Survival data

Specific techniques are required for the analysis of clinical trials when the main evaluation of patient outcome is whether the patient does or does not 'fail' (where, for example, failure is 'death' or 'relapse') and information is available on the time from entry into the trial until failure. The statistical analysis of such data, called survival data, is discussed in Chapter 14, pp. 210–216.

Protocol

This is a written document outlining the purposes of the clinical study including the rationale, the method of administering the treatments and the details concerning the plan of investigation. A successful trial is dependent on the validity of its protocol. The format of the protocol depends on individual taste. As a *guideline*, the protocol might contain details pertaining to:

1. Introduction and rationale for the trial, including references.
2. Objectives.

3. Design.

4. Criteria for inclusion and exclusion of patients and a confirmation (or otherwise) of their consent.

5. Procedures in the event of response, no response, side-effects, drop-outs and defaulters.*

6. Treatment programmes.

7. Methods and frequency of assessments.

8. Statistical considerations.

9. Record forms.

10. Study chairman and responsible investigators.

Note: Consideration must be given as to whether patients withdrawn from treatment, for whatever reason, should be included in the analysis of results. In most circumstances, all patients, including these *withdrawals* (provided their evaluation continues throughout the study) should be included in the analysis. The rationale behind this decision depends on the distinction between the *explanatory* approach (aimed at understanding under 'laboratory' conditions) and the *pragmatic* approach (aimed at decision under 'normal' conditions) to clinical trials. This distinction is relevant to many aspects of the conduct and analysis of clinical trials (such as the form in which treatments are provided, the constitution of patient groups, the criteria for assessing outcome as well as the handling of drop-outs). It forms the basis of, and is discussed at length in Schwartz, D., Flamant, R. and Lellouch, J. (1980) *Clinical Trials,* Academic Press.

Chapter 14
Vital Statistics

Introduction

Two areas closely allied with medical statistics are:

1. *Demography*—the study of human populations, providing information about the distributions of characteristics (such as age, sex, race, geographic distribution and occupation) in these populations.
2. *Epidemiology*—the study of the distribution and determinants of disease frequency in populations. Its main aims are to provide data for medical planning and to acquire knowledge of *causal* mechanisms that can form a basis for preventive measures against diseases and for the study of biological processes such as multiple pregnancies and fertility.

Although statistical methodology is used extensively in demography and epidemiology, it is not the function of this text to provide a comprehensive account of these topics. The reader is referred to Fleiss, J. (1981) and MacMahon, B. and Pugh, T. F. (1970) for full discussions.

However, some consideration (principally of a statistical nature) is given to *vital statistics* and to *observational studies* (e.g. to evaluate the effects of vaccination, screening, fluoridation of water, etc.). These topics are included because of their inherent statistical methodology and because *vital statistics* and their analysis are fundamental to the study of demography and epidemiology and *observational studies* comprise the bulk of epidemiological research.

Definition

Vital statistics is the body of knowledge encompassing the study of census and registration data such as that relating to birth, death and illness.

Rates

In this chapter, attention is confined to morbidity, fertility, mortality and survival, each of which may be measured by a *rate*. A rate pertaining to an event (e.g. death) has the following components:

1. The number of events occurring.
2. The period of occurrence of these events. This may not be the unit time interval (e.g. 1 year) in which the rate is expressed.
3. The population at risk; i.e. the number of people to whom these events could occur: conventionally, the number in the population at the midpoint of the time interval (rather than the average number).
4. A convenience factor, C, which allows the rate to be expressed in a form which is easily assimilated. Multiplying the rate per unit of population, usually a small fraction, by C (often $C = 100\,000$ or 1000) produces a rate per C of population which is a larger, more manageable number.

A rate of occurrence of an event per C of the population per unit time is of the general form:

$$\text{Rate} = \frac{\text{Number of events per unit time}}{\text{Number in population at risk}} \times C.$$

Occasionally a rate (e.g. birth rate) does not conform precisely to this definition because the denominator of the ratio does not strictly refer to the population at risk. For practical purposes, all such ratios are called rates.

The rate is called a *crude* rate if none of the factors which may affect the rate (e.g. age, sex, social class, etc.) are taken into account.

The rate is called a *specific* rate if it relates to a particular section (e.g. sex, occupation, age group) of the population.

Measures of morbidity (sickness)

1. Total sickness = number of persons sick.
2. Incidence rate

$$= \frac{\begin{array}{c}\text{Number of illnesses or spells of illness } \textit{beginning}\text{; or number} \\ \text{of persons } \textit{becoming} \text{ sick in a specified period of time}\end{array}}{\text{Number exposed to risk at midpoint of period}}.$$

3. Period prevalence rate

$$= \frac{\text{Number of illnesses, spells of illness or sick persons existing } \textit{at any time} \text{ within a specified period of time}}{\text{Number exposed to risk at midpoint of period}}.$$

4. Point prevalence rate

$$= \frac{\text{Number of illnesses, spells of illnesses or sick persons existing at a } \textit{specified point in time}}{\text{Number exposed to risk at that point in time}}.$$

5. Average duration of sickness $= \dfrac{\text{Point prevalence rate}}{\text{Incidence rate}}$:

a. Per person

$$= \frac{\text{Total number of days of illness in a defined period}}{\text{Number exposed to risk at midpoint of the period}} \times C.$$

b. Per sick person

$$= \frac{\text{Total number of days of illness in a defined period}}{\text{Number of sick people during the period}} \times C.$$

c. Per illness

$$= \frac{\text{Total number of days of illness in a defined period}}{\text{Number of spells of sickness during the period}} \times C.$$

Fertility and mortality (death) rates

1. Birth rate $= \dfrac{\text{Number of live births in a year}}{\text{Mid-year population}} \times C.$

2. Fertility rates:

a. Total

$$= \frac{\text{Number of live-births in a year}}{\text{Mid-year population of women aged 15–44}} \times C.$$

b. Legitimate

$$= \frac{\text{Number of legitimate live-births in a year}}{\text{Mid-year population of married women aged 15–44}} \times C.$$

c. Illegitimate

$$= \frac{\text{Number of illegitimate live-births in a year}}{\text{Mid-year population of single, widowed and divorced women aged 15–44}} \times C.$$

3. Infant mortality rate

$$= \frac{\text{Number of deaths under 1 year in a year}}{\text{Number of live-births in the year}} \times C.$$

4. Neonatal mortality rate

$$= \frac{\text{Number of deaths under 4 weeks in a year}}{\text{Number of live-births in the year}} \times C.$$

5. Stillbirth rate

$$= \frac{\text{Number of stillbirths in a year}}{\text{Total of births (live+still) in the year}} \times C.$$

6. Perinatal mortality rate

$$= \frac{\text{Number of stillbirths and deaths under 1 week in a year}}{\text{Total number of births (live+still) in the year}} \times C.$$

7. Maternal mortality rate

$$= \frac{\text{Number of deaths from puerperal causes in a year}}{\text{Total number of confinements in the year}} \times C.$$

Sometimes the last three rates are calculated with total live-births only in the denominator.

8. Proportional mortality rate

$$= \frac{\text{Number of deaths in a given age group (or from a given cause) in a year}}{\text{Total number of deaths in the year}} \times C.$$

Usually the proportional mortality rate is expressed as a percentage in which case $C = 100$.

9. Crude mortality rate $= \dfrac{\text{Number of deaths in a year}}{\text{Mid-year population}} \times C.$

10. Standardised mortality rate = an average death rate in which allowance is made for (generally) the age and sex composition of the population. It is a fictitious rate useful for comparative purposes.

Methods of standardising mortality rates

There are two main ways of deriving standardised rates: (i) direct method; and (ii) indirect method.

Direct method

1. Define a standard population.
2. For each age–sex stratum, multiply the age–sex specific death rate of the index population (the population under consideration) by the number of individuals in the equivalent age–sex stratum of the standard population. This product is the expected number of deaths in the standard population for that age–sex stratum.
3. Add the expected number of deaths in the standard population in all the age–sex strata.
4. The *standardised death rate* (SDR) is the crude death rate for these expected deaths, i.e.

$$\text{SDR} = \frac{\text{Total number of expected deaths in the standard population}}{\text{Number in the standard population}} \times C.$$

Note: The *comparative mortality index* (CMI) is obtained by dividing this standardised death rate by the crude rate of the standard population.

Requirements: A knowledge for each age–sex stratum of the index population of: (i) the number of individuals in the stratum; and (ii) the number of deaths in the stratum.

Indirect method

1. Define a standard set of specific rates.
2. For each age–sex stratum, multiply the standard age–sex specific mortality rate by the number of individuals in the equivalent age–sex stratum of the index population. This product is the expected number of deaths in the index population for that age–sex stratum.
3. Add the expected number of deaths in the index population in all the age–sex strata.
4. The *standardised mortality ratio* (SMR) is often used as an index of relative mortality without further calculations and is given by

$$\text{SMR} = \frac{\text{Total deaths observed in the index population}}{\text{Total deaths expected in the index population}} \times C.$$

5. Standardised death rate

    = SMR×Crude death rate of the standard population

$$= \text{SMR} \times \frac{\text{Number of deaths in the standard population}}{\text{Number in the standard population}} \times C.$$

Advantages of the indirect method: (i) Requires no knowledge of the specific rates of the index population; and (ii) when the index population is small, it is not necessary to use rates calculated from a small number of events.

Life tables

The life table shows the number of persons who, of a given number (the *radix*, usually chosen to be a convenient quantity such as 1000) born or living at a specified age, live to attain successive higher ages, together with the numbers who die in the interval.

The tables may be: (i) *Full*—every single year of age is included from 0 to the highest age to which any person survives; or (ii) *abridged*—the ages are considered in groups (e.g. 5 year age groups). Often the first few years of life are examined singly.

There are two types of table:

1. The *current life table* describes the survival pattern of a group of individuals subject throughout life to the age–sex specific mortality rates observed at one point in time. It summarises current mortality and may be used as an alternative to methods of standardisation to compare the mortality patterns of different populations.

2. The *cohort life table* describes the actual survival experience of a group or cohort of individuals born at the same time. It summarises the mortality of the cohort at different ages at the times when the individuals in the cohort are at these ages. Cohort life tables are particularly useful in studies of occupational mortality.

Uses of the life table

1. To summarise the *mortality patterns* experienced by a specified population subjected to certain age specific mortality rates, permitting a useful comparison with other populations.

2. To investigate the distribution of *survival times* in *follow-up studies* of patients after some critical event such as appearance of symptoms, admission to hospital, completion of a prescribed form of treatment, etc. Such a life table relates the numbers living and dying to the length of time since the critical event rather than to the age of the individual. In other respects, its composition is similar to the life table described below.

Content of the current life table

The life table contains the following columns:

Column 1, x

The age (starting at 0) in single years (full life table) or in groups of years (abridged life table) to which the numbers in the other columns relate.

Column 2, d_x

The number of individuals who die in the interval x to $x+1$ ($x+1$ is the next age or age group, as applicable, after x).

Column 3, $n_x = n_{x-1} - d_{x-1}$

The number of individuals alive at the start of the interval x.

Column 4, $q_x = d_x/n_x$

The probability that an individual, alive at the start of the interval x, will die in the interval, i.e. will not be alive at the start of the interval $x+1$.

Note: (i) If the life table is used in a follow-up study of survival, some account should be taken of the 'withdrawals', w_x, i.e. the patients lost to follow-up. Assuming they are evenly spread over the interval, an adjustment is made to the denominator, n_x (in $q_x = d_x/n_x$), by replacing it by $n'_x = n_x - w_x/2$. (ii) If the age specific death rate of the interval, m_x, is available, it is unnecessary to include the columns d_x and n_x in the life table, since q_x may be calculated directly from the identity $q_x = (2m_x)/(2+m_x)$.

Column 5, $p_x = 1-q_x$

The probability that an individual, alive at the start of the interval x, will survive to the next interval.

Column 6, $l_x = l_0 p_0 p_1 \cdots p_{x-1}$

The number of individuals out of an arbitrary l_0 (the radix which is usually 100 for follow-up studies, 1000 or 1000000) born alive who would survive to the start of the interval x.

Note: (i) If the life table is used in a follow-up study of survival and $l_0 = 100$, then l_x gives the *life table survival rate*, l_x being the percentage of survivors after x years. (ii) It can be shown (see Armitage, P. (1987), p. 427) that the approximate variance of l_x is given by

$$\text{Var}(l_x) \simeq l_x^2 \sum_{i=0}^{x-1} \frac{d_i}{n_i'(n_i'-d_i)}$$

If l_x is assumed to be approximately normally distributed, approximate 95% confidence limits for the true value of l_x are $l_x \pm 1.96 \sqrt{\text{Var}(l_x)}$.

Column 7, $e_x = (l_{x+1}+l_{x+2}+\ldots)/l_x+1/2$

The expectation of life at age x; i.e. the average additional length of life lived by those l_x individuals alive at the start of the interval x. It is generally assumed the deaths are evenly spread over the interval.

Note: The expectation of life is not calculated from follow-up studies unless the period of follow-up is sufficiently long to cover the complete span of survival. This is rare.

Survival data

Survival data contains information about the time taken for individuals to reach a defined end-point, often called a *failure* (e.g. death, recurrence of disease, etc.). In each individual, this failure can occur at most once, and may not occur at all in the course of the study. When there is incomplete observation of the failure time (i.e. the patient is still alive at the time of analysis if the failure is 'death') then the data are said to be *censored*. For convenience, failure is represented by 'death' in the remainder of this section. Then the failure time is an indicator of survival experience (hence the terminology) which forms the basis of clinical trials into potentially fatal chronic diseases (e.g. cancer).

The techniques of survival data analysis are only outlined in this text as the subject is relatively complex. The reader is referred to Oakes, D. (1983), pp. 305–11, and Anderson, S. *et al.* (1980), pp. 199–234 for essentially non-technical accounts, and to Karlbfleisch, J. D. and Prentice, R. L. (1980) for a fuller discussion.

Survival data can be analysed in various ways. The following procedures may be of interest:

1. Construction of survival curves.

A life-table or actuarial survival curve is concerned with the distribution of survival times in a single group. The information is most easily assimilated by a graphical representation, called a *survival curve*, in which the horizontal axis typically represents the time elapsed from the start of the investigation, and the vertical axis designates the percentage of individuals surviving. Two approaches to estimating the survival curve are methods due to:

a. *Berkson and Gage*—the technique is appropriate when survival times are grouped into intervals and the number of individuals dying in each interval is recorded (i.e. the current life-table technique (pp. 209–210) replacing age, x, by survival time, t).

b. *Kaplan–Meier*—the analysis is based on precise survival times rather than on grouped data. See Matthews, D. E. and Farewell, V. (1985), pp. 69–78 for a description, and to the Examples section of this chapter.

2. Comparison of two (or more) survival curves.

A comparison of survival curves is relevant when each curve differs with respect to a certain factor, such as treatment. Essentially, its purpose is to determine whether the failure times are longer in one group compared to the other(s). Three common approaches to the problem are:

a. The data are *dichotomised according to survival or non-survival* for a given critical period after entry, typically 5 years, and crude survival rates are calculated.

The *advantages* of this approach are:
   (i) simplicity,
   (ii) by analysing contingency tables it allows a quantitative assessment of the effect of explanatory variables.
The major *disadvantages* are:
   (i) it wastes information as it concentrates only on a single point in time.

(ii) it is not appropriate when the data are censored.

b. The survival times are *not assumed to follow any known distribution* and methods based on life-table calculations are used. In particular:

(i) TWO ESTIMATED SURVIVAL RATES for a given critical period of time, t, after entry, each obtained from a separate life-table, can be compared using a standardised normal deviate (see Colton, T., 1974, p 249). In the life-table described on pp. 208–210, the age, x, is replaced by the survival time, t, so that l_x is replaced by the estimated survival rate, $l(t)$, which is assumed to be approximately normally distributed. This approach is generally inefficient as only part of the information in each life-table is used.

(ii) THE LOG-RANK (OR MANTEL–HAENSZEL) TEST can be performed to test the null hypothesis that the survival curves are the same. This test compares the number of deaths observed in each treatment group with the number of deaths expected if the two (or more) treatments are equally effective. The log-rank test involves:

(A) determining the numbers of observed and expected deaths at each death time (i.e. at each point in time at which a death occurs),

(B) summing these quantities, appropriately, to evaluate the total numbers of observed and expected deaths in each treatment group (i.e. O_i and E_i, respectively, in treatment group i ($i = 1, 2, \ldots, k$),

(C) comparing the survival curves, under the null hypothesis that they are identical, by calculating a test statistic [containing the totals mentioned in (B), above] whose distribution is approximately chi-square with $k-1$ degrees of freedom. In particular, if $k = 2$, then the test statistic is

$$(O_1 - E_1)^2/E_1 + (O_2 - E_2)^2/E_2.$$

Note: The log-rank test can be adapted to compare the survival experience of individuals receiving different treatments when *adjustments are made for prognostic factors*, provided these factors are qualitative (i.e. can be categorised). The patients are divided into subgroups or strata defined by the prognostic factors (e.g. sex, age categories). The calculations of observed and expected numbers of deaths for a log-rank test are performed within each stratum. The test statistic is computed from values of O_i and E_i $(i = 1, 2, \ldots, k)$ which are obtained by summing the respective observed and expected values from all the strata. Care must be taken to retain a moderate number of patients within each stratum if this approach to adjusting for prognostic factors is to be effective. Thus stratification is generally limited to at most eight strata unless the study is very large, and is probably most effective with up to four strata.

The reader is referred to Peto, R. *et al.* (1977) for a full discussion of the log-rank test, and to the Examples section of this chapter for an illustration of the technique.

c. The survival times are assumed to follow a *known distribution*, commonly the *exponential*, although other possibilities include the Weibull, the log-normal and the Gamma distributions.

Some terms must be explained before the exponential distribution of survival times can be defined. In general, the *hazard function*, $\lambda(t)$, is the time dependent risk of failure (i.e. the probability of failing at a specified time, t, when it is known that the individual did not fail before t). When the failure is 'death', the hazard function may be thought of as an instantaneous death rate, and it is sometimes called the *force of mortality*.

If there is a *time independent risk of death* (i.e. the hazard function is *constant* over time) so that $\lambda(t) = \lambda$, then the survivor function, $l(t)$, is

$$\Pr(\text{survival} > t) = \exp(-\lambda t)$$

and t is said to follow an *exponential* distribution with mean survival time, $1/\lambda$.

An empirical check of the *appropriateness of the exponential model* for a set of survival data is provided by constructing the life-table, estimating the survivor function, $l(t)$, from it and then plotting $\log_e l(t)$ versus t. Such a plot should approximate a straight line with slope, $-\lambda$.

If the exponential model is appropriate then the death rate, λ, can be estimated by

$$\hat{\lambda} = \frac{\text{number of deaths}}{\text{total follow-up time}}$$

whose logarithm is approximately normally distributed with variance $1/d$, where d is the observed number of deaths.

Two exponential survival curves can be compared by calculating the ratio of two estimated failure rates, and testing their significance by taking logarithms and determining the appropriate standardised normal deviate. The reader is referred to Healy, M. J. R. and Osborn, J. (1986), pp. 173–182 for details, and to the Examples section of this chapter. *Note:* The ratio of these rates is equivalent to the relative risk discussed in Chapter 15.

3. Formulation of particular regression models.

Survival data may be analysed by constructing a suitable regression model which incorporates censoring and allows for the simultaneous influence of a number of *explanatory or predictor variables*. These variables can be qualitative or quantitative and may measure demographic properties (e.g. sex, age on entry to the study) or describe medical history, etc.

PROPORTIONAL HAZARD FUNCTIONS

When the hazard function is constant over time (see **2(c)** above), the survival times follow an exponential distribution, and a comparison of two survival curves by estimating their relative risk is quite a simple procedure. When the hazard function for each group depends on time, it may be reasonable to assume that the *hazard functions are proportional*, i.e. for each time, t,

$$\lambda_1(t) = \theta\lambda_0(t)$$

where $\lambda_i(t)$ = hazard function for treatment $i(i = 0, 1$, where, typically, $i = 0$ for the control or standard group and $i = 1$ for the treatment group).

There are various procedures for estimating the ratio of hazard functions (the relative risk), θ, in these circumstances.

CONFOUNDING FACTIONS

In addition, the comparison between treatment groups may be distorted by confounding factors. Fortunately, the proportional hazards model can easily be extended to include the effects of these factors.

Suppose $\underline{x} = (x_1, x_2, \ldots, x_k)$ is an observed set of explanatory variables representing treatment (e.g. $x_1 = 0$ and $x_1 = 1$ specify two treatment groups) and prognostic factors. Let $\lambda(t, \underline{x})$ be the death rate (hazard function) at time t for an individual with observed values of the explanatory variable, $\underline{x}$. Let $\lambda_0(t)$ be a reference point representing the death rate at time t for an individual in the standard population whose covariate values are all zero. Then *Cox's proportional hazard's model* specifies that

$$\lambda(t, \underline{x}) = \lambda_0(t) \exp \sum_{i=1}^{k} \beta_i x_i$$

i.e. the death rate for an individual with covariate values $\underline{x}$ is a constant multiple, $\exp \sum \beta_i x_i$, of the baseline death rate (i.e. that of the standard population) at all times. The ratio of these two rates is equivalent to the relative risk (see Chapter 15, p. 230).

Alternatively, by taking logarithms, the model can be written as

$$\log_e \lambda(t, \underline{x}) = \log_e \lambda_0(t) + \sum_{i=1}^{k} \beta_i x_i$$

which is the familiar multiple regression equation with the constant term, a, being replaced by $\log_e \lambda_0(t)$, a function of time. It can be seen that this model is similar to the multiple logistic regression equation (see Chapter 11, pp. 153–154) with the odds ratio being replaced by a rate ratio.

ANALYSIS

The *regression coefficients*, β_1, β_2, $\ldots$, β_k, in the proportional hazards model can be estimated by b_1, b_2, $\ldots$, b_k, respectively, with their standard errors using a suitable computer program based on the method of maximum likelihood. These coefficients indicate the extent to which the death rate is affected by treatment and prognostic factors. If $\beta_i = 0$ $(i = 1, 2, \ldots, k)$ then the associated covariate is not related to survival when adjustment is made for the other covariates included in the model. A positive coefficient, β_i, indicates that the log hazard function increases with x_i so that high values of x_i are associated with poorer survival. If $c_i = \exp(\beta_i)$, then c_i is the multiplicative effect of the variable x_i. For example, suppose x_2 represents sex such that $x_2 = 0$ for males and $x_2 = 1$ for females. Then c_2 is what the rate for males must be multiplied by to give the rate for females, all other things being equal. Furthermore, the relative risk for an individual with covariate values, $\underline{x}$, is estimated by $\exp \sum b_i x_i$.

The reader is referred to Osborn, J. F. (1986), pp. 63–64, for a simple discussion of the proportional hazards model.

Examples

Methods of standardising mortality rates

The standardised death rates are required for Hospitals A and B (Table E14.1).

Direct method

1. Define the total cases in the two hospitals together as the standard population.

Table E14.1 Mortality from a given disease in two hospitals over a period of several years

Age group (years)	Hospital A			Hospital B			Hospital (A+B)		
	Cases	Deaths	Rate per 1000 cases	Cases	Deaths	Rate per 1000 cases	Cases	Deaths	Rate per 1000 cases
0–4	128	32	250	93	27	290	221	59	267
5–9	573	46	80	325	27	83	898	73	81
10–14	429	40	93	300	27	90	729	67	92
15–19	397	42	106	317	35	110	714	77	108
⩾ 20	201	35	174	186	30	161	387	65	168
Total	1728	195	113	1221	146	120	2949	341	116

Source: Hypothetical data.

2. The expected number of deaths in an age stratum in the standard population is found by multiplying the death rate of the stratum in Hospital A by the number of cases in the equivalent age stratum in the standard population [e.g. $55.3 = (221)(250)/(1000)$, $71.8 = (898)(80)/(1000)$, etc.]. The procedure is repeated using the cases in Hospital B as the index population. The results are presented in Table E14.2.

3. The expected number of deaths in the standard population, using the cases in Hospital A as the index population, are summed

Table E14.2 Expected deaths in the standard population [i.e. Hospitals (A+B)]

Age groups (years)	Cases in standard population	Expected deaths in standard population using rates from:	
		A	B
0–4	221	55.3	64.1
5–9	898	71.8	74.5
10–14	729	67.8	65.6
15–19	714	75.7	78.5
≥ 20	387	67.3	62.3
Total	2949	337.9	345.0

Source: Table E14.1.

to give the total expected number of deaths. The total expected number of deaths is similarly determined when the cases in Hospital B form the index population. The results are presented in Table E14.2.

4. SDR for A $= \dfrac{337.9}{2949} \times 1000 = 114.6$.

SDR for B $= \dfrac{345.0}{2949} \times 1000 = 117.0$.

Note: Crude rate for population $= \dfrac{341}{2949} = 115.6$.

CMI for A $= \dfrac{114.6}{115.6} = 0.99$.

CMI for B $= \dfrac{117.0}{115.6} = 1.01$.

Indirect method

1. Define the age-specific rates in Hospitals (A+B) as the standard set of rates.

2. The expected number of deaths in an age stratum of Hospital A is found by multiplying the death rate of the stratum in the standard population by the number of cases in the equivalent age stratum in Hospital A [e.g. 34.2 = (267/1000)(128), etc.]. The procedure is repeated using the cases in Hospital B as in index population. The results are presented in Table E14.3.

Table E14.3 Expected deaths with combined rates

Age group (years)	Cases in population		Expected deaths	
	A	B	A	B
0–4	128	93	34.2	24.8
5–9	573	325	46.4	26.3
10–14	429	300	39.5	27.6
15–19	397	317	42.9	34.2
⩾ 20	201	186	33.8	31.2
Total	1728	1221	196.8	144.1

Source: Table E14.1.

3. The expected number of deaths are summed to give the total expected number of deaths in Hospitals A and B. The results are presented in Table E14.3.

4. SMR for A $= \dfrac{195}{196.8} = 0.99$.

SMR for B $= \dfrac{146}{144.1} = 1.01$.

5. SDR for A $= (0.99)\left(\dfrac{341}{2949}\right) = 114.5$.

SDR for B $= (1.01)\left(\dfrac{341}{2949}\right) = 116.8$.

Life tables

Table E14.4 shows the life table calculations for patients suffering from carcinoma of the oesophagus. All patients were admitted to the hospitals in a district between 1970 and 1974 and discharged after radical oesophagectomy. They were followed up each year to 31 December, 1975. Unfortunately, some patients were lost to follow-up because they moved from the district. It is assumed that these patients are an unselected group who left the district uniformly throughout the year.

Table E14.4 Life table for patients after radical oesophagectomy

Interval since operation (years) $x-$	Deaths in interval d_x	Losses to follow-up w_x	No. alive at start of interval n_x	Adjusted no. at risk n'_x	Estim. prob. of death q_x	Estim. prob. of survival p_x	Percentage of survivors after x years l_x
0–	17	10	207	202.0	0.0842	0.9158	100
1–	26	3	180	178.5	0.1457	0.8543	91.6
2–	33	0	151	151.0	0.2185	0.7815	78.2
3–	28	6	118	115.0	0.2435	0.7565	61.1
4–	21	2	84	83.0	0.2530	0.7470	46.3

Source: Hypothetical data.

Survival data

Kaplan–Meier survival curves and the log-rank test

Suppose it is of interest to compare the survival experience in two groups of patients, i.e. those patients receiving treatments A or B, randomly (see Peto, R. *et al.*, 1977). The trial time is derived for each of 25 patients from details of the date of randomisation and the date of death if the patient died before the follow-up date of 31 May, 1974. The survival times (days from randomisation), arranged in ascending order for each treatment group, are presented in Table E14.5 together with a statement of the number of deaths at each survival time. Clearly, the data are censored in that some patients are still alive at the time of analysis.

The *Kaplan–Meier survival curves* are estimated using the data in Table E14.5. It should be noted that:

1. For convenience, an initial row of the table is defined, indicating that the estimated percentage of survivors beyond day 0 is 100%.
2. In each treatment group in this study, the patients still alive have longer survival times than the patients who have died. Thus the censored data can be ignored, and the percentage of survivors after t days estimated simply as

$$\frac{\text{numbers of patients surviving beyond } t}{\text{total number of patients}} \times 100\%.$$

Table E14.5 Tabulation for Kaplan–Meier survival curves

	Treatment Group						
	A				B		
Survival time, t (days)	No. deaths on day t	% survivors after t days* (a)	% survivors after t days* (b)	Survival time, t (days)	No. deaths on day t	% survivors after t days* (a)	% survivors after t days* (b)
0	0	$(12/12)100$	$= 100$	0	0	$(13/13)100$	$= 100$
8	2	$(10/12)100$	$= [10/(10+2)]100 = 83.3$	13	1	$(12/13)100$	$= [12/(12+1)]100 = 92.3$
52	1	$(9/12)100$	$= [9/(9+1)]83.3 = 75.0$	18	1	$(11/13)100$	$= [11/(11+1)]92.3 = 84.6$
63	2	$(7/12)100$	$= [7/(7+2)]75.0 = 58.3$	23	1	$(10/13)100$	$= [10/(10+1)]84.6 = 76.9$
220	1	$(6/12)100$	$= [6/(6+1)]58.3 = 50.0$	70	1	$(9/13)100$	$= [9/(9+1)]76.9 = 69.2$
365	0			76	1	$(8/13)100$	$= [8/(8+1)]69.2 = 61.5$
852	0			180	1	$(7/13)100$	$= [7/(7+1)]61.5 = 53.8$
1296	0			195	1	$(6/13)100$	$= [6/(6+1)]53.8 = 46.2$
1328	0			210	1	$(5/13)100$	$= [5/(5+1)]46.2 = 38.5$
1460	0			632	1	$(4/13)100$	$= [4/(4+1)]38.5 = 30.8$
1976	0			700	1	$(3/13)100$	$= [3/(3+1)]30.8 = 23.1$
				1296	1	$(2/13)100$	$= [2/(2+1)]23.1 = 15.4$
				1990	0		
				2240	0		

Source: Peto, R., Pike, M. C., Armitage, P. *et al.* (1977) Design and analysis of randomised clinical trials requiring prolonged observation of each patient: II analysis and examples. *Br. J. Cancer*, **35**, 1–39.

*See text for distinction between the calculations of columns (a) and (b).

An alternative expression for the estimated percentage of survivors after t days, appropriate whether or not the data are censored, is

$$\frac{\text{number of patients surviving beyond } t}{\text{number surviving beyond } t + \text{number dying at } t} \times \begin{pmatrix} \text{est. \% survivors} \\ \text{after previous} \\ \text{survival time} \end{pmatrix} \%$$

$$= \begin{array}{l} \text{estimated probability of surviving day } t \times \\ \text{for those alive at start of day } t \end{array} \begin{pmatrix} \text{estimated \%} \\ \text{surviving up to} \\ \text{day } t \end{pmatrix} \%$$

The resultant Kaplan–Meier survival curves are shown in Fig. E14.1.

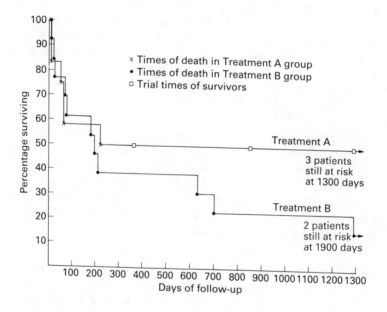

Fig. 14.1 Kaplan–Meier survival curves for the data of Table E14.5.

Two methods are evolved to compare the survival experience in the two treatment groups. One method is based on the assumption that the data are approximately exponentially distributed in each group, and the other makes no distributional assumptions and is the log-rank test.

1. As the data appear, by inspection of Fig. E14.1, to be approximately **exponentially** distributed in each treatment group, the survival curves are compared initially by considering the estimated mortality rates, $\hat{\lambda}_i = d_i/(\text{total follow-up time in group } i)$ where d_i = number of deaths in group i, and $i = A, B$.

Then

$$\hat{\lambda}_A = 5/6491 = 7.703 \times 10^{-4} \text{ per day.}$$
$$\hat{\lambda}_B = 12/8921 = 1.345 \times 10^{-3} \text{ per day.}$$

The ratio of these two rates, the estimated relative risk, is

$$\hat{R} = \hat{\lambda}_A/\hat{\lambda}_B = 0.57.$$

It can be shown that $\log_e \hat{\lambda}_i$ is approximately normally distributed with variance $1/d_i$. Thus the standardised normal deviate to test the significance of the ratio of the true mortality rates, R, from unity (or, equivalently, that of $\log_e R = \log_e \lambda_A - \log_e \lambda_B$ from zero) is

$$\frac{\log_e \hat{\lambda}_A - \log_e \hat{\lambda}_B}{\sqrt{[(1/d_A) + (1/d_B)]}} = \frac{-0.5575}{0.5323} = -1.047$$

which, referring to Table A1, is not significant, $P > 0.05$.

Furthermore, the 95% confidence limits for $\log_e R$ are $-0.5575 \pm 1.96(0.5323) = -1.6008$ and 0.4858. Thus the limits for R are $\exp(-1.6008)$ and $\exp(0.4858) = -0.20$ and 1.63.

It should be noted that this test is more efficient than the nonparametric log-rank test described below if the assumption of exponential survival times is valid.

2. a. Although the data appear to be approximately exponentially distributed in each group, it is considered a useful exercise to perform a **log-rank test** to compare the survival experience in the two treatment groups. The data necessary for this calculation are presented in Table E14.6, in which the patients are arranged in order of increasing trial time (if there is a tie, the patients who died on that day are listed before the patients who did not). From Table E14.6, the following results are obtained:

O_A = observed number of deaths in Group A = 6
E_A = expected number of deaths in Group A = 8.34
O_B = observed number of deaths in Group B = 11
$E_B = (O_A + O_B) - E_A = 17 - 8.34 = 8.66$.

Table E14.6 Details of the log-rank test calculations and of renal function

Trial time, t, days	Treatment	Death during trial time Y = Yes N = No	d_t	n_t	n_{At}	n_{Bt}	$e_{At} = \dfrac{n_{At}\, d_t}{n_t}$	Renal function I = impaired N = normal
8 ⎱	A	Y	2	25	12	13	0.960	I
8 ⎰	A	Y						N
13	B	Y	1	23	10	13	0.435	I
18	B	Y	1	22	10	12	0.435	I
23	B	Y	1	21	10	11	0.476	I
52	A	Y	1	20	10	10	0.500	I
63 ⎱	A	Y	2	19	9	10	0.947	I
63 ⎰	A	Y						I
70	B	Y	1	17	7	10	0.412	N
70	B	Y	1	16	7	9	0.438	N
180	B	Y	1	15	7	8	0.467	N
195	B	Y	1	14	7	7	0.500	N
210	B	Y	1	13	7	6	0.538	N
220	A	Y	1	12	7	5	0.583	N
365	A	N	0	11	6	5	0.000	N
632	B	Y	1	10	5	5	0.500	N
700	B	Y	1	9	5	4	0.556	N
852	A	N	0	8	5	3	0.000	N
1296 ⎱	B	Y	1	7	4	3	0.571	N
1296 ⎰	A	N						N
1328	A	N	0	5	3	2	0.000	N
1460	A	N	0	4	2	2	0.000	N
1976	A	N	0	3	1	2	0.000	N
1990	B	N	0	2	0	2	0.000	N
2240	B	N	0	1	0	1	0.000	N
Total			17				$E_A = 8.338$	

Source: Peto, R., Pike, M.C., Armitage, P. *et al*. (1977) Design and analysis of randomised clinical trials requiring prolonged observation of each patient: II analysis and examples. *Br. J. Cancer*, **35**, 1–39.

t = number of days a patient is observed.
d_t = number of deaths during day t.
n_t = overall number at risk on day t.
n_{At} = number at risk on day t in Group A.
n_{Bt} = number at risk on day t in Group B.
e_{At} = extent of exposure to risk in Group A on day t
   = conditional expected number of deaths in Group A on day t.

Note: E_B can be calculated as the difference between the total number of observed deaths $(O_A + O_E)$ and E_A, and so values of $e_{Bt} = n_{Bt} d_t / n_t$ do not have to be calculated separately for each trial time and then summed to produce E_B.

Then

$$X^2 = (O_A - E_A)^2 / E_A + (O_B - E_B)^2 / E_B$$

with a calculated value of

$$X_C^2 = 1.29.$$

Referring to the table of the χ^2 distribution (Table A2) with 1 degree of freedom, $P > 0.05$. This suggests that the apparent superiority of treatment A could well have arisen by chance alone.

b. Suppose that, in addition, the **relevance of renal function to prognosis** is to be investigated (see last column of Table E14.6). The log-rank test can be adapted when *adjustments are made for this prognostic factor*. The patients are divided into two subgroups according to whether their renal function is impaired or normal. Then the calculations of observed and expected numbers of deaths for a log-rank test within each subgroup are performed. The results are presented in Table E14.7.

Table E14.7 Observed and expected numbers of deaths by treatment and renal function

| | | Treatment | | | |
| | | A | | B | |
		Observed deaths	Expected deaths	Observed deaths	Expected deaths
Renal	Impaired	4	5.42	3	1.58
function	Normal	2	5.01	8	4.99
	Total	6	10.43	11	6.57

X^2 is determined as before except that the renal function adjusted total numbers of expected deaths are used instead of E_A and E_B. It is calculated as

$$X^2_{AC} = (6 - 10.43)^2 / 10.43 + (11 - 6.57)^2 / 6.57$$
$$= 4.87.$$

Referring to the table of the χ^2-distribution (Table A2) with one degree of freedom, $0.025 < P < 0.05$, i.e. the difference in prognosis between the two treatment groups, once an adjustment is made for renal function, is statistically significant, although only marginally so.

Note: The relative death rate in Group A is 0.58 (i.e. 6/10.43) and that in Group B is 1.67 (i.e. 11/6.57) after an adjustment is made for the effects of renal condition on the extent of exposure to risk of death. Thus the ratio of the death rate on Treatment A to that on Treatment B is 0.34 (i.e. 0.58/1.67), i.e. the death rate observed on A is about 1/3 of that on B.

Chapter 15
Observational Studies

Experimental *vs* observational studies

Epidemiological studies may be broadly classified as experimental or non-experimental (i.e. observational) studies. An *experimental* study, investigating a cause–effect relationship, generally relies on the deliberate reduction in a natural exposure or application of a preventive measure, and inspection of the subsequent appearance, or lack of it, of the effect. The opportunities for experimental studies in human populations are quite rare. Thus, in this test, attention is confined to *observational studies* which investigate cause–effect relationships by observing events in their natural setting without recourse to experimental intervention.

Case-control *vs* cohort studies

Two types of observational study aimed at accumulating sufficient knowledge about the aetiology of a disease to generate preventative measures for it are:

1. *Case-control studies*—in which groups of individuals with (the cases) and without (the controls) the disease are selected and compared with respect to those characteristics (risk factors) thought to be relevant to the aetiology of the disease.

2. *Cohort studies*—in which the groups of individuals (the cohorts) to be studied are classified according to characteristics of interest and are observed over a period of time. Then rates of occurrence of various manifestations of disease can be determined and related to the classifications by aetiological factors. The period of study time relative to the investigator's place in time, and hence the ensuing cohort study, may be:

    a. *Retrospective*—all the relevant events (exposures to risk as well as effects) have already occurred when the study is initiated, and the data are obtained from existing records.

    b. *Prospective*—the cohorts are defined by potential aetiological factors at the start of the investigation, and are followed forward in time until the various manifestations of disease are observed in the individuals. Most cohort studies are prospective.

Note: Case-control studies are sometimes called retrospective studies because they involve looking backward from effects to preceding causes. By analogy, *cohort* studies are sometimes called prospective studies because they involve looking forward from causes to effects. The author prefers to use the terms 'case-control' and 'cohort' studies in these contexts.

Cross-sectional *vs* longitudinal studies

An additional characterisation of epidemiological studies depends on the time-span separating the agents of cause and effect. In particular, in a:

1. *Longitudinal* study—the observations on cause and effect relate to two different points in time, even if they are collected simultaneously. Most cohort and case-control studies are longitudinal.
2. *Cross-sectional* study—the observations on cause and effect relate to a single point in time. Such studies are limited to those in which the causal mechanisms are relatively permanent characteristics of the individual. Cross-sectional studies may provide evidence of association between factors of interest, but, because they do not involve time, cannot elucidate causation. However, cross-sectional studies are easier and more economical than longitudinal studies.

Case-control studies

Advantages

1. Generally inexpensive.
2. Can be completed in a relatively short period of time because:
  a. both case and control groups can be selected quite quickly (except for the study of rare diseases)
  b. it may be easy to obtain information concerning exposure to possible aetiological factors.
3. Can simultaneously evaluate many causal hypotheses.
4. Permits the evaluation of interaction—the extent and manner

in which two (or more) causes of disease modify the strength of one another.

5. Applicable to rare as well as common diseases.

6. By describing incidence rates of disease according to various risk factors at a point in time, they provide a 'picture' of the disease in a population.

7. Permit evaluation of causal significance.

Disadvantages

1. They are susceptible to several sources of bias such as those relating to the:

    a. Comparability of cases and controls with respect to the history of risk factor exposure. For example, (i) from records, when the risk factor often occurs artificially more frequently amongst the cases than the controls, because it is looked for and recorded more often in the former group; or (ii) from personal interviews when information is subject to memory failure, to faulty interpretation of the questions by the interviewees or to the answers by the interviewer, or to extensive probing amongst the cases.

    b. Selection of controls and their comparability with the cases. Even when cases and controls are matched with respect to possible aetiological variables, other unidentified variables, differing in the two groups, may influence the findings.

    c. Selection of cases and the identification of risk factors. Physicians may differ in the criteria they apply for diagnosing disease. The diagnosis of disease may be influenced by the presence of risk factors. Furthermore, the definition of risk factors is sometimes imprecise and can lead to discrepancies.

    d. Fact that individuals with both the disease and the factor may be more likely to be included in the study than those who have only one or the other. This would result in a spuriously high frequency of risk factors amongst the cases, and is an example of Berkson's fallacy; see Colton, T. (1974), pp. 305–309.

2. If there is an association between a risk factor and a disease, then the magnitude of the increase in disease risk brought about by the factor's presence cannot be estimated directly. However, it is possible to obtain an indirect estimate of the relative risk (see below, unmatched cases and controls, measure of association, Note 1).

Analysis of case-control studies

The basic approach to the analysis of a case-control study of the aetiological effect of some factor on a disease involves comparing the proportion of cases who are exposed to the factor with the proportion of controls who are exposed. Interest is centred on assessing the statistical significance of the observed differences as well as measuring the disparity between the apparent risks of the disease in those with and without the factor.

Two situations must be distinguished, namely when the cases and controls are *matched* and when they are *unmatched*. Generally the controls are individually matched to the cases with respect to any known or potential confounding variables to enable the aetiological factors under investigation to be assessed independently of these variables.

Unmatched cases and control

Suppose two *independent* samples of n_1 cases and n_2 controls are selected. The number of individuals in each group exposed to the suspected aetiological factor is determined and the results are arranged in a fourfold table; see Table 15.1.

Table 15.1 Observed frequencies of individuals relating their disease status to factor exposure

	Disease		
	Present, D+ (Cases)	Absent, D− (Controls)	Total
Factor — Present, F+ (exposed)	a	b	$m_1 = a+b$
Factor — Absent, F− (unexposed)	c	d	$m_0 = c+d$
Total	$n_1 = a+c$	$n_0 = b+d$	$n = a+b+c+d$
Proportion exposed	$p_1 = a/n_1$	$p_0 = b/n_0$	

1. Statistical test of association

An approximate test of association in a fourfold table is the chi-square test (see pp. 119–120). It tests the statistical significance of the difference between the proportions exposed to the factor in the groups with (cases) and without (controls) the disease. Using the notation of Table 15.1, the test statistic is

$$X_Y^2 = \frac{n(|ad-bc|-n/2)^2}{n_1 n_0 m_1 m_0}$$

whose sampling distribution is χ^2 with one degree of freedom.

2. Measure of association

A measure of the strength of the association between the disease and the exposure to the factor is the *relative risk*. The relative risk, R, is usually taken as the ratio of disease rates (generally incidence or mortality) in the exposed and unexposed portions of the population. It is estimated in the case-control study by $\hat{R} = (ad)/(bc)$.

Notes

1. Case-control studies are orientated towards the computation of *exposure rates to the factor* amongst diseased and non-diseased individuals. The relative risk is derived from *disease rates* amongst individuals exposed, and not exposed to the factor. Hence, the relative risk *cannot be estimated directly* in case-control studies. However, under the assumptions that (i) the disease under study is relatively infrequent in exposed and unexposed individuals, and (ii) neither cases nor controls are selected in favour of either exposed or non-exposed individuals, then the above *indirect* estimate of relative risk, $\hat{R}$, can be obtained for R, and is a useful index of association even if the above assumptions do not hold.

2. For a *justification* of $\hat{R}$ as an estimate of R, see MacMahon, B. and Pugh, T. F. (1970), pp. 270–273.

3. $\hat{R}$ is often called the relative odds or the *odds ratio* (see also Chapter 11, p. 154). It is the ratio of affected to unaffected individuals in one group divided by the same ratio in another group.

4. $\log_e \hat{R}$ has approximately a normal distribution with an estimated variance (Vâr) for large samples of

$$\text{Vâr}(\log_e \hat{R}) \simeq 1/a + 1/b + 1/c + 1/d.$$

Confidence limits can be obtained for $\log_e R$ (and, therefore, for R by taking antilogs) in the usual way using normal theory. For example, approximate 95% confidence limits for $\log_e R$ are

$$\log_e \hat{R} \pm 1.96 \sqrt{\text{Vâr}(\log_e \hat{R})}.$$

5. ½ is sometimes added to each cell of the observed frequency table if it contains zero entries to avoid dividing by zero when estimating R and its variance.

6. Sometimes it is of interest to *compare* and, if appropriate, *combine* estimates of relative risk obtained from different studies or from different subgroups of the population (e.g. different age groups). The entries in the ith of a series of k 2×2 tables are identified in Table 15.2.

Table 15.2 Observed frequencies of individuals in the ith 2×2 table ($i = 1$, $2, \ldots, k$)

		Disease		
		Present (Cases)	Absent (Controls)	Total
Factor	Present	a_i	b_i	m_{1i}
	Absent	c_i	d_i	m_{0i}
Total		n_{1i}	n_{0i}	n_i

a. *Comparison of k relative risks*
An appropriate test statistic to test the null hypothesis that the k relative risks, estimated by $\hat{R}_i (i = 1, 2, \ldots, k)$, are equal is

$$\sum_{i=1}^{k} w_i y_i^2 - \left(\sum_{i=1}^{k} w_i y_i \right)^2 \bigg/ \left(\sum_{i=1}^{k} w_i \right)$$

whose distribution is approximately χ^2 with $k-1$ degrees of freedom, where, for the ith subgroup ($i = 1, 2, \ldots, k$)

$$y_i = log_e \hat{R}_i$$
$$w_i = 1/[\text{Vâr}(y_i)]$$
$$\text{Vâr}(y_i) \simeq 1/a_i + 1/b_i + 1/c_i + 1/d_i$$

using the notation of Table 15.2.

b. *Combination of k estimates of relative risk*
If the result of the above test (from **a**) is not significant, the k estimates of relative risk may be combined to produce a pooled estimate. The *Mantel–Haenszel* estimate of the true relative risk is often used and is given by

$$\hat{R}_{MH} = \left(\sum_{i=1}^{k} W_i \hat{R}_i \right) \bigg/ \left(\sum_{i=1}^{k} W_i \right) = \left(\sum_{i=1}^{k} a_i d_i / n_i \right) \bigg/ \left(\sum_{i=1}^{k} b_i c_i / n_i \right)$$

where $W_i = b_i c_i / n_i$ and $\hat{R}_i = (a_i d_i)/(b_i c_i)$, i.e. it is a weighted average of the estimated relative risks.

The approximate 95% confidence limits for the true relative risk are given by

$$\hat{R}_{MH}^{(1 \pm 1.96/S)}$$

where S^2 is defined below.

See Mantel, N. and Haenszel, W. (1959), pp. 719–748, for a full discussion.

c. *Test of the null hypothesis that there is no association in all tables (Mantel–Haenszel test)*
The test statistic,

$$S^2 = \frac{\left(\left| \sum_{}^{k} a_i - \sum_{}^{k} n_{1i} m_{1i}/n_i \right| - \frac{1}{2} \right)^2}{\sum_{}^{k} \{ (n_{1i} n_{0i} m_{1i} m_{0i})/[n_i^2(n_i - 1)] \}},$$

is used to test the null hypothesis that the relative risk in every table (a pooled estimate of which is the Mantel–Haenszel estimate) is unity. The distribution of S^2 is approximately χ^2 with one degree of freedom.

See Breslow, N. E. and Day, N. E. (1980), pp. 136–143, for a full discussion of Note **6**.

Matched cases and controls

When the controls are individually matched to the cases, then the subsequent analysis should take the pairings into account. The observed frequencies of pairs are usually presented in a two-way table, of the general form of Table 15.3.

Table 15.3 Observed frequencies of pairs of individuals

Controls (disease absent, D−)	Cases (disease present, D+)	
	Factor present (F+)	Factor absent (F−)
Factor present (F+)	r	s
Factor absent (F−)	t	u

1. Statistical test of association
An approximate test of association when the two samples consist

of paired individuals is McNemar's test (see pp. 120–123). In this context, it tests the null hypothesis that the proportions of individuals exposed to the factor are the same in the groups with (cases) and without (controls) the disease (or, alternatively, that the expectations of s and t are equal). Using the notation of Table 15.3, the test statistic is

$$T_3^2 = (|s-t|-1)^2/(s+t)$$

whose sampling distribution is χ^2 with one degree of freedom. The (-1) in the numerator is a correction factor which is often ignored. It should be remembered that the analysis is based solely on *untied* pairs, i.e., on those pairs in which one member is exposed and the other is not exposed to the factor under study.

2. Measure of association

The strength of the association between the disease and the exposure to the factor is usually measured by the relative risk. In this situation the true relative risk is estimated by

$$\hat{R}_M = t/s.$$

Approximate 95% confidence limits for the true relative risk are given by

$$\hat{R}_M^{(1\pm1.96/T_3)}$$

See Miettinen, O. S., 1970, pp. 75–86, for a full discussion, and also pp. 235–236, for an analogous justification.

Cohort studies

Attention is centred on prospective cohort studies as these are most common.

Advantages

The advantages of cohort studies are that:

1. The comparability of the two groups (i.e. those with and without the risk factor) can be determined at the start of the investigation. It is often possible to identify variables for which adjustments will be necessary in the analysis, and to plan the analysis accordingly.

2. Information concerning exposure to the risk factor is usually current at the time it is elicited. Thus the criteria for establishing the presence of the risk factor can be established uniformly, and the recording of exposure to the risk factor is less subject to mis-classification than in the case-control study.

3. As cohort studies generally proceed from present to future time, they permit criteria for future identification of disease to be established uniformly.

4. The scope of measurement is more versatile in a cohort study than in a case-control study. The former does not rely so heavily on information contained in records, with their inherent disadvantages. However, there is no recovery from failure to include a key variable at the outset of a cohort study.

5. Disease occurrence can be expressed as an incidence rate. The difference between these rates in exposed and unexposed groups provides a *direct* estimate of the magnitude of increased risk.

Disadvantages

The disadvantages of cohort studies are that:

1. Studies are large, particularly for rare diseases.

2. They are time-consuming, as long periods of follow-up may be required before sufficient number of cases develop or if there is a long latency of effect.

3. Good follow-up presents a major difficulty because (i) individuals may move away or refuse to participate, and (ii) the enthusiasm of the investigators may wane over time. Particular difficulties arise when termination of follow-up is related to the development of the disease.

4. They are generally expensive.

5. An important limiting factor is the difficulty of selecting comparison groups which are representative of the exposed and unexposed segments of a *general* population. Usually nonrepresentative but available populations (e.g. physicians) are used, and the generalisation of their results to wider populations is not a matter of statistics but rather of judgement.

Analysis of cohort studies

The analysis of data from cohort studies involves the derivation of disease rates, and their comparison between various exposure groups of the same cohort or between exposed and non-exposed cohorts. These comparisons are generally achieved by estimating the *relative risk* (see p. 230).

The process of estimating this risk depends on the data available. The relative risk can be estimated *directly* in a *cohort* study in which disease rates amongst exposed and non-exposed individuals can be elicited. *Note*: The relative risk can only be estimated indirectly in case-control studies which are orientated towards the computation of exposure rates to the factor amongst diseased and non-diseased individuals.

In cohort studies, consideration must be given to whether the relative risk is defined as the ratio of two proportions or two rates.

1. Proportions—the true disease rate in the exposed group is the proportion of individuals in the exposed population with the disease (i.e. the ratio of the number of individuals with the disease in the exposed population to the number exposed). Similarly, for the unexposed group. No account is taken of the duration of observation of each individual.

2. Rates—a frequently used denominator for calculating rates of the specified outcome (such as disease) is person–years (person–weeks or whatever) of observation. This denominator takes simultaneously into consideration the number of persons under observation and the duration of observation of each person. Then the disease rate in the exposed group is the ratio of the number of individuals in the exposed group with the disease to the person–years (say) at risk in the exposed group.

The estimates of relative risk, with their estimated variances, test statistics and approximate confidence limits are given in Table 15.4.

Notes

1. Since the distributions of $\hat{R}_1$ and $\hat{R}_2$ are approximately normal, both of the test statistics, S_1 and S_2, for testing the null hypothesis that the true relative risk is unity (or equivalently, that its logarithm is zero) are standardised normal deviates. The significance of each is determined by referring to Table A1.

2. The approximate 95% confidence limits for R_i (often called Miettinen's test based confidence limits) are derived from the approximate 95% confidence limits for $\log_e R_i (i = 1, 2)$. These are

$$\log_e \hat{R}_i \pm 1.96 \sqrt{\text{V}\hat{\text{a}}\text{r}(\log_e \hat{R}_i)} = \log_e \hat{R}_i \pm 1.96 \log_e \hat{R}_i / S_i$$
$$= \log_e \hat{R}_i [1 + 1.96/S_i].$$

Table 15.4 Relative risk in cohort studies

	Disease rate expressed as ratio of two	
	proportions $(i = 1)$	rates $(i = 2)$
Estimated relative risk, $\hat{R}_i$	$\dfrac{p_e}{p_o} = \dfrac{r_e}{n_e} \Big/ \dfrac{r_o}{n_o}$	$\dfrac{m_e}{m_o} = \dfrac{r_e}{n'_e} \Big/ \dfrac{r_o}{n'_o}$
Est. variance $\text{Vâr}(\log_e \hat{R}_i)$	$\dfrac{1-p_e}{r_e} + \dfrac{1-p_o}{r_o}$	$\dfrac{1}{r_e} + \dfrac{1}{r_o}$
Test statistic, S_i, for $H_0: R_i = 1$	$\dfrac{\log_e \hat{R}_1}{\sqrt{\{[(1-p_e)/r_e]+[(1-p_o)/r_o]\}}}$	$\dfrac{\log_e \hat{R}_2}{\sqrt{[(1/r_e)+(1/r_o)]}}$
Approximate 95% confidence limits for R_i	$\hat{R}_1^{1 \pm 1.96/S_1}$	$\hat{R}_2^{1 \pm 1.96/S_2}$

where, in the exposed and unexposed samples, respectively:
(1) r_e and r_o are the number of diseased individuals
(2) n_e and n_o are the number of individuals
(3) n'_e and n'_o are the person–years at risk
(4) m_e and m_o are the disease rates.

Thus the approximate 95% confidence limits for R_i are

$$\exp[\log_e \hat{R}_i(1 \pm 1.96/S_i)] = \hat{R}_i^{1 \pm 1.96/S_i}$$

Examples

Case-control studies—unmatched cases and controls

Tuyns, A. J. *et al* (1977), pp. 45–60, report the results of a study of 200 males diagnosed with oesophageal cancer in one of the regional hospitals between January 1972 and 1974. Controls were a sample of 775 adult males drawn from electoral lists in each commune. Tuyns *et al* were interested in investigating the relationship between alcohol consumption and the risk of oesophageal cancer. Table E15.1. summarises the data for alcohol consumption, dichotomised at a value of 80 g/day for cases and controls.

1. Statistical test of association
The test statistic is

$$X_Y^2 = \frac{n(|ad-bc|-n/2)^2}{n_1 n_0 m_1 m_0}$$

Table E15.1   2×2 table relating average daily alcohol consumption to disease status

		Disease status		
		Cases (D+)	Controls (D−)	Total
Average daily	≥ 80	96	109	205
alcohol consumption (g)	< 80	104	666	770
Total		200	775	975
Percentage (≥ 80 g)%*		48.00	14.06	21.03

Source: Tuyns, A. J. *et al.* (1977) Le cancer de l'oesophage en Ille-et-Vilaine en fonction des niveaux de consommation d'alcool et de tabac. *Bull. Cancer,* **64,** 45–60.
*These are the observed percentages of individuals with an averege daily alcohol consumption of ≥ 80 g.

$$X^2_{YC} = \frac{975(|(96)(666)-(109)(104)|-975/2)^2}{(205)(770)(200)(775)}$$

$$= 108.1.$$

From the table of the χ^2 distribution (Table A2), $\chi^2_1(0.001) = 10.83$. Hence $X^2_{YC} > \chi^2_1(0.001)$. Thus there is evidence of an association between alcohol consumption and disease status, $P < 0.001$.

2. Measure of association

The relative risk is estimated by

$$\hat{R} = \frac{ad}{bc} = \frac{(96)(666)}{(109)(104)} = 5.64.$$

The estimated variance of its logarithm is

$$\begin{aligned}
\text{Vâr}(\log_e \hat{R}) &\simeq 1/a + 1/b + 1/c + 1/d \\
&= 1/96 + 1/109 + 1/104 + 1/666 \\
&= 0.0307.
\end{aligned}$$

Note: Using these estimates, an alternative test statistic for the test of association (**1**, above), testing that R is unity or, equivalently, that $\log_e R$ is zero, is given by $\log_e \hat{R}/\sqrt{[\text{Vâr}(\log_e \hat{R})]} = (1.730)/\sqrt{(0.0307)} = 9.87$ whose distribution is approximately normal. Referring to Table A1, $P < 0.001$, as above.

Approximate 95% confidence limits for $\log_e R$ are given by $\log_e 5.64 \pm 1.96\sqrt{(0.0307)} = 1.730 \pm 0.343 = 1.387$ and 2.073. Thus the approximate 95% confidence limits for the true relative risk, R, are given by $\exp(1.387)$ and $\exp(2.073) = 4.00$ and 7.95.

Since the incidence rates of most cancers rise sharply with age, Tuyns *et al* were particularly interested in investigating the association of alcohol consumption with disease status in *different age groups*. Table E15.2 divides the population into six 10-year age intervals, yielding a series of 2×2 tables whose sum is the single 2×2 table, Table E15.1.

3. Comparison of six relative risks

To test the null hypothesis that the six relative risks, estimated by $\hat{R}_i (i = 1, 2, \ldots, 6)$, are equal, the test statistic is

$$\sum w_i y_i^2 - (\sum w_i y_i)^2 / (\sum w_i) = 80.539 - (45.609)^2 / (28.261)$$
$$= 6.933,$$

whose distribution is approximately χ^2 with 5 degrees of freedom. Referring to Table A2, $P > 0.05$.

4. Combination of six relative risks

Since the result of the above test is not significant, the *Mantel–Haenszel* pooled estimate of relative risk is calculated. It is given by

$$\hat{R}_{MH} = \left(\sum_{i=1}^{6} a_i d_i / n_i \right) \Big/ \left(\sum_{i=1}^{6} b_i c_i / n_i \right) = (58.439)/(11.330) = 5.158$$

i.e. after adjusting for the effect of age, the relative risk is estimated by 5.16. (*Note:* $\hat{R}_{MH} = 5.16$ is slightly lower than the value of $\hat{R} = 5.64$ obtained without stratification by age.) Approximate confidence limits for R_{MH} are given by

$$\hat{R}_{MH}^{(1 \pm 1.96/S)} = 5.158^{(1 \pm 1.96/9.122)}$$
$$= 5.158^{(0.785)} \text{ and } 5.158^{(1.215)}$$
$$= 3.62 \text{ and } 7.34$$

where

$$S^2 = \frac{\left(\left| \sum_{i=1}^{k} a_i - \sum_{i=1}^{k} n_{1i} m_{1i} / n_i \right| - \frac{1}{2} \right)^2}{\sum_{i=1}^{k} \{ (n_{1i} n_{0i} m_{1i} m_{0i}) / [n_i^2 (n_i - 1)] \}}$$

so that its calculated value is

$$S_C^2 = \frac{(|96 - 48.890| - \frac{1}{2})^2}{26.106}$$
$$= 83.22$$

and $\qquad\qquad S_C = 9.122.$

Table E15.2 2×2 tables relating average daily alcohol consumption to disease status for six strata defined by 10-year age intervals

Stratum i	Age (years)	Average daily alcohol consumption (g)	Disease status Case	Control	Odds ratio $\hat{R}_i = \frac{a_i d_i}{b_i c_i}$	$y_i = \log_e \hat{R}_i^*$	$w_i = [\hat{Var}(\log_e \hat{R}_i)]^{-1}$†	$\frac{a_i d_i}{n_i}$	$\frac{b_i c_i}{n_i}$	$\frac{n_{1i} m_{1i}}{n_i}$	$\frac{n_{1i} n_{0i} m_{1i} m_{0i}}{n_i^2(n_i-1)}$
1	25–34	≥ 80	1	9	∞	3.515	0.360	0.914	0.328	0.086	0.079
		< 80	0	106							
2	35–44	≥ 80	4	26	5.05	1.625	2.233	3.296	0.653	1.357	1.106
		< 80	5	164							
3	45–54	≥ 80	25	29	5.67	1.717	7.884	16.197	2.859	11.662	6.858
		< 80	21	138							
4	55–64	≥ 80	42	27	6.36	1.832	10.412	24.124	3.793	21.668	10.670
		< 80	34	139							
5	65–74	≥ 80	19	18	2.58	0.938	6.943	10.385	4.025	12.640	6.449
		< 80	36	88							
6	≥ 75	≥ 80	5	0	∞	3.708	0.429	3.523	0.0	1.477	0.944
		< 80	8	31							
Total			96	109			28.261	58.439	11.330	48.890	26.106
			104	666							

Source: Tuyns, A. J. *et al.* (1977) Le cancer de l'oesophage en Ille-et-Vilaine en fonction des niveaux de consommation d'alcool et de tabac. *Bull. Cancer*, **64**, 45–60.

* ½ is added to each cell to avoid the value ∞ resulting from dividing by zero. An alternative approach would be to combine sub-tables 1 and 2 (corresponding to strata levels) and sub-tables 5 and 6.

† $\hat{Var}(\log_e \hat{R}_i) = 1/a_i + 1/b_i + 1/c_i + 1/d_i$.

5. Test of the null hypothesis that there is no association in all tables (Mantel–Haenszel test)
The test statistic is calculated as

$$S_C^2 = 83.22 \quad \text{(see above)}$$

whose distribution is approximately χ^2 with one degree of freedom. Referring to Table A2, $P < 0.001$. Thus there appears to be evidence of an association between alcohol consumption and the risk of oesophageal cancer, with an age-adjusted relative risk, R_{MH}, estimated by 5.16. The approximate 95% confidence limits for R_{MH} are 3.62 and 7.34.

Case-control studies—matched cases and controls

A retrospective case-control study was undertaken to examine the association between endometrial carcinoma and the use of oestrogens in post-menopausal women (see Osborn, J. F. (1986), pp. 71–73). There were 317 cases and 317 matched controls from the same hospital. The matching criteria were age at diagnosis and year of diagnosis. The 317 controls were patients with cervical carcinoma, ovarian cancer or carcinoma of the vulva.

Table E15.3 shows the distribution of pairs of individuals categorised according to whether each patient had taken oestrogens for at least 6 months prior to the diagnosis of cancer, or had not taken oestrogens.

1. Statistical test of association (McNemar's test)
The test statistic is

$$T_3^2 = \frac{(|s-t|-1)^2}{s+t}$$

$$T_{3C}^2 = \frac{(|15-113|-1)^2}{15+113} = 73.51$$

whose distribution is approximately χ^2 with one degree of freedom. Referring to the table of the χ^2 distribution (Table A2), $P < 0.001$, i.e. there is evidence of an association between endometrial carcinoma and the use of oestrogens in post-menopausal women.

2. Measure of association
The relative risk is estimated by

$$\hat{R}_M = \frac{t}{s} = \frac{113}{15} = 7.53$$

Table E15.3 Observed frequencies of 317 pairs of post-menopausal women

| | Cases | | |
	Oestrogen used	Oestrogen not used	Total
Controls			
Oestrogen used	39	15	54
Oestrogen not used	113	150	263
Total	152	165	317

Source: Osborn, J. F. (1986) *Basic Statistical Methods for Epidemiological Studies*. London: London School of Hygiene and Tropical Medicine.

i.e. there is nearly an eightfold increase in the risk of endometrial carcinoma brought about by taking oestrogens.

The approximate 95% confidence interval for the true relative risk is given by

$$\hat{R}_M^{1 \pm 1.96/T_3} = 7.53^{1 \pm 1.96/8.57}$$
$$= 4.75 \text{ to } 11.95.$$

3. Effect of ignoring the matching

If the matching of cases and controls is ignored, Table E15.4 (derived from Table E15.3) adequately presents the results.

The relative risk, ignoring matching, is estimated by

$$\hat{R} = \frac{(152)(263)}{(54)(165)} = 4.49$$

Table E15.4 2×2 table relating use of oestrogens to disease status

| | Disease status | |
	Cases (D+)	Controls (D−)
Oestrogens used	152	54
Oestrogens not used	165	263
Total	317	317

Source: Table E15.3.

with approximate 95% confidence limits for R given by $\exp\{\log_e(4.49)\pm1.96\sqrt{[\text{Vâr}(\log_e \hat{R})]}\} = \exp(1.5019\pm0.3667) = 3.11$ and 6.48, where $\text{Vâr}(\log_e \hat{R}) \simeq /(152)+1/(54)+1/(165)+1/(263) = 0.0305$. i.e. this estimate of relative risk ($\hat{R} = 4.49$) is less than the estimate obtained when the information concerning the matching of cases and controls is used ($\hat{R}_M = 7.53$). In general, ignoring the matching has the effect of introducing a bias to the estimate of relative risk, bringing it closer to the null value of unity.

Analysis of cohort studies

1. Proportions

A randomised double-blind multicentre clinical trial was performed to determine whether continuation of well-controlled oral anti-coagulant (AC) therapy, in elderly patients who had received this therapy ever since their primary myocardial infarction (MI), would result in a major decrease in total mortality over a period of 2 years (see Report of the Sixty Plus Reinfarction Study Research Group, 1980, pp. 989–994). Half of the 878 patients, all over 60 years of age, received placebos instead of the AC, the others continued AC therapy. All were followed for 2 years.

The mortality observed for the two groups is shown in Table E15.5. The estimated relative risk of death is

$$\hat{R}_1 = \frac{p_e}{p_o} = \frac{28}{439} \Big/ \frac{49}{439} = 0.57$$

$$\text{Vâr}(log_e \hat{R}_1) = \frac{1-p_e}{r_e}+\frac{1-p_o}{r_o}$$

$$= 0.05157.$$

Test statistic for testing the null hypothesis that the relative risk is unity is

$$S_1 = \frac{\log_e \hat{R}_1}{\sqrt{\{[(1-p_e)/r_e]+[(1-p_o)/r_o]\}}}$$

with a calculated value of

$$S_{1C} = -2.46.$$

Referring $|S_{1C}|$ to Table A1, $P = 0.014$

Table E15.5 Distribution of deaths within 2 years in two groups of patients, those 'exposed' to AC(*e*) and an unexposed placebo group (*o*)

	Placebo	AC	Total
Number dead	49	28	77
Number alive	390	411	811
Total	439	439	878
Proportion dead	0.112	0.064	0.088

Source: Report of the Sixty Plus Reinfarction Study Research Group (1980) A double-blind trial to assess long-term oral anticoagulant therapy in elderly patients after myocardial infarction. *Lancet* **ii**, 989–994.

Approximate 95% confidence limits for R_1 are

$$\hat{R}_1^{1\pm1.96/S_1} = 0.57^{1\pm(-0.7954)}$$
$$= 0.57^{1.7954} \text{ and } 0.57^{0.2046}$$
$$= 0.36 \text{ and } 0.89.$$

Table E15.6 Relative risk of nonfatal MI and fatal CHD by categories of parental history

	Nonfatal MI Parental history		Fatal CHD Parental history	
	None (*o*)	≤ 60 (*e*)	None (*o*)	≤ 60 (*e*)
Cases	75	40	17	16
Person–years	304,203	59,386	330,997	64,275
Rate, m_e		6.74×10^{-4}		2.49×10^{-4}
Rate, m_o	2.47×10^{-4}		5.14×10^{-5}	
$\hat{R}_2 = m_e/m_o$	2.73		4.85	
Vâr($\log_e \hat{R}_2$)	0.038		0.121	
Test statistic, S_2	5.13 ($P < 0.001$)		4.53 ($P < 0.001$)	
95% conf. limits for $\hat{R}_2$	1.86 and 4.01		2.53 and 9.59	

Source: Colditz, G. A. *et al.* (1986) A prospective study of parental history of myocardial infarction and coronary heart disease in women. *Am. J. Epidemiol.* **123**, 43–58.

Thus there was a significant ($P < 0.05$) relative risk of death of 0.57 (approximate 95% confidence limits 0.36 and 0.89) in the AC group compared to the placebo group.

2. Rates

A prospective study among 117156 US women, free from coronary heart disease (CHD) and aged 30–55 years in 1976, was conducted to investigate the impact of parental myocardial infarction (MI) on the incidence of CHD (see Colditz *et al.* 1986, pp. 48–58). The women completed questionnaires in 1976 from which information on parental history and other risk factors was elicited. Questionnaires in 1978 and 1980 identified women who had developed nonfatal MI. Fatal CHD cases were ascertained by searches of state vital records. The women were followed until June 1, 1980.

The number of person–years of follow-up differed for the two end-points. Since the whole cohort was followed for fatal outcomes, all the person–years of the cohort were used for fatal CHD. Since nonfatal events were ascertained from the returned questionnaires, the person–years for questionnaire respondents were used for nonfatal MI. The results for those women who reported no parental history of MI and a parental history of MI $\leq$ 60 years of age are shown in Table E15.6 (in which the notation and formulae used correspond to those in Table 15.4). Clearly, there was an increased risk of both nonfatal MI and fatal CHD for women with a parental history of MI $\leq$ 60 years of age compared to those with no family history.

Appendix
Statistical Tables

Table A1 Percentage points of the standard normal distribution

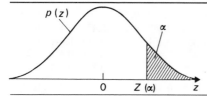

The percentage point, $Z(\alpha)$, beyond which lies $100\alpha\%$ of the total probability is tabulated for various values of α. The distribution is symmetric about $Z(0.50) = 0$ so that $Z(\alpha) = -Z(1-\alpha)$.

	3rd decimal place of α									
α	0.000	0.001	0.002	0.003	0.004	0.005	0.006	0.007	0.008	0.009
0.00	∞	3.090	2.878	2.748	2.652	2.576	2.512	2.457	2.409	2.366
0.01	2.326	2.290	2.257	2.226	2.197	2.170	2.144	2.120	2.097	2.075
0.02	2.054	2.034	2.014	1.995	1.977	1.960	1.943	1.927	1.911	1.896
0.03	1.881	1.866	1.852	1.838	1.825	1.812	1.799	1.787	1.774	1.762
0.04	1.751	1.739	1.728	1.717	1.706	1.695	1.685	1.675	1.665	1.655
0.05	1.645	1.635	1.626	1.616	1.607	1.598	1.589	1.581	1.572	1.563
0.06	1.555	1.546	1.538	1.530	1.522	1.514	1.506	1.499	1.491	1.483
0.07	1.476	1.468	1.461	1.454	1.447	1.440	1.433	1.426	1.419	1.412
0.08	1.405	1.398	1.392	1.385	1.379	1.372	1.366	1.360	1.353	1.347
0.09	1.341	1.335	1.329	1.323	1.317	1.311	1.305	1.299	1.293	1.287
0.10	1.282	1.276	1.270	1.265	1.259	1.254	1.248	1.243	1.237	1.232
0.11	1.227	1.221	1.216	1.211	1.206	1.200	1.195	1.190	1.185	1.180
0.12	1.175	1.170	1.165	1.160	1.555	1.150	1.146	1.141	1.136	1.131
0.13	1.126	1.122	1.117	1.112	1.108	1.103	1.099	1.094	1.089	1.085
0.14	1.080	1.076	1.071	1.067	1.063	1.058	1.054	1.049	1.045	1.041
0.15	1.036	1.032	1.028	1.024	1.019	1.015	1.011	1.007	1.003	0.999
0.16	0.995	0.990	0.986	0.982	0.978	0.974	0.970	0.966	0.962	0.958
0.17	0.954	0.950	0.946	0.942	0.939	0.935	0.931	0.927	0.923	0.919
0.18	0.915	0.912	0.908	0.904	0.900	0.897	0.893	0.889	0.885	0.882
0.19	0.878	0.874	0.871	0.867	0.863	0.860	0.856	0.852	0.849	0.845
0.20	0.842	0.838	0.835	0.831	0.827	0.824	0.820	0.817	0.813	0.810
0.21	0.806	0.803	0.800	0.796	0.793	0.789	0.786	0.782	0.779	0.776
0.22	0.772	0.769	0.766	0.762	0.759	0.755	0.752	0.749	0.745	0.742
0.23	0.739	0.736	0.732	0.729	0.726	0.723	0.719	0.716	0.713	0.710
0.24	0.706	0.703	0.700	0.697	0.694	0.690	0.687	0.684	0.681	0.678

Table A1 *continued*

α	0.000	0.001	0.002	0.003	0.004	0.005	0.006	0.007	0.008	0.009
				3rd decimal place of α						
0.25	0.675	0.671	0.668	0.665	0.662	0.659	0.656	0.652	0.650	0.646
0.26	0.643	0.640	0.637	0.634	0.631	0.628	0.625	0.622	0.619	0.616
0.27	0.613	0.610	0.607	0.604	0.601	0.598	0.595	0.592	0.589	0.586
0.28	0.583	0.580	0.577	0.574	0.571	0.568	0.565	0.562	0.559	0.556
0.29	0.553	0.551	0.548	0.545	0.542	0.539	0.536	0.533	0.530	0.527
0.30	0.524	0.522	0.519	0.516	0.513	0.510	0.507	0.504	0.502	0.499
0.31	0.496	0.493	0.490	0.487	0.485	0.482	0.479	0.476	0.473	0.471
0.32	0.468	0.465	0.462	0.459	0.457	0.454	0.451	0.448	0.445	0.443
0.33	0.440	0.437	0.434	0.432	0.429	0.426	0.423	0.421	0.418	0.415
0.34	0.413	0.410	0.407	0.404	0.402	0.399	0.396	0.393	0.391	0.388
0.35	0.385	0.383	0.380	0.377	0.375	0.372	0.369	0.367	0.364	0.361
0.36	0.359	0.356	0.353	0.351	0.348	0.345	0.343	0.340	0.337	0.335
0.37	0.332	0.329	0.327	0.324	0.321	0.319	0.316	0.313	0.311	0.308
0.38	0.306	0.303	0.300	0.298	0.295	0.292	0.290	0.287	0.285	0.282
0.39	0.279	0.277	0.274	0.272	0.269	0.266	0.264	0.261	0.259	0.256
0.40	0.253	0.251	0.248	0.246	0.243	0.240	0.238	0.235	0.233	0.230
0.41	0.228	0.225	0.222	0.220	0.217	0.215	0.212	0.210	0.207	0.205
0.42	0.202	0.199	0.197	0.194	0.192	0.189	0.187	0.184	0.182	0.179
0.43	0.176	0.174	0.171	0.169	0.166	0.164	0.161	0.159	0.156	0.154
0.44	0.151	0.148	0.146	0.143	0.141	0.138	0.136	0.133	0.131	0.128
0.45	0.126	0.123	0.121	0.118	0.116	0.113	0.111	0.108	0.106	0.103
0.46	0.100	0.098	0.095	0.093	0.090	0.088	0.085	0.083	0.080	0.078
0.47	0.075	0.073	0.070	0.068	0.065	0.063	0.060	0.058	0.055	0.053
0.48	0.050	0.048	0.045	0.043	0.040	0.038	0.035	0.033	0.030	0.028
0.49	0.025	0.023	0.020	0.018	0.015	0.013	0.010	0.008	0.005	0.003

Condensed from Table 4 of Pearson, E. S. and Hartley, H. O. (1966) *Biometrika Tables for Statisticians,* 3rd Edn. Cambridge: Cambridge University Press.

Table A2 Percentage points of the χ^2 distribution

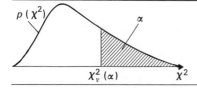

The percentage point, $\chi_v^2(\alpha)$, beyond which lies $100\alpha\%$ of the total probability, is tabulated for various values of v and α (DF, degrees of freedom).

DF	0.975	0.900	0.750	0.500	α 0.250	0.100	0.050	0.025	0.010	0.001
1	—	0.02	0.10	0.45	1.32	2.71	3.84	5.02	6.63	10.83
2	0.05	0.21	0.58	1.39	2.77	4.61	5.99	7.38	9.21	13.82
3	0.22	0.58	1.21	2.37	4.11	6.25	7.81	9.35	11.34	16.27
4	0.48	1.06	1.92	3.36	5.39	7.78	9.49	11.14	13.28	18.47
5	0.83	1.61	2.67	4.35	6.63	9.24	11.07	12.83	15.09	20.52
6	1.24	2.20	3.45	5.35	7.84	10.64	12.59	14.45	16.81	22.46
7	1.69	2.83	4.25	6.35	9.04	12.02	14.07	16.01	18.48	24.32
8	2.18	3.49	5.07	7.34	10.22	13.36	15.51	17.53	20.09	26.12
9	2.70	4.17	5.90	8.34	11.39	14.68	16.92	19.02	21.67	27.88
10	3.25	4.87	6.74	9.34	12.55	15.99	18.31	20.48	23.21	29.59
11	3.82	5.58	7.58	10.34	13.70	17.28	19.68	21.92	24.72	31.26
12	4.40	6.30	8.44	11.34	14.85	18.55	21.03	23.34	26.22	32.91
13	5.01	7.04	9.30	12.34	15.98	19.81	22.36	24.74	27.69	34.53
14	5.63	7.79	10.17	13.34	17.12	21.06	23.68	26.12	29.14	36.12
15	6.27	8.55	11.04	14.34	18.25	22.31	25.00	27.49	30.58	37.70
16	6.91	9.31	11.91	15.34	19.37	23.54	26.30	28.85	32.00	39.25
17	7.56	10.09	12.79	16.34	20.49	24.77	27.59	30.19	33.41	40.79
18	8.23	10.86	13.68	17.34	21.60	25.99	28.87	31.53	34.81	42.31
19	8.91	11.65	14.56	18.34	22.72	27.20	30.14	32.85	36.19	43.82
20	9.59	12.44	15.45	19.34	23.83	28.41	31.41	34.17	37.57	45.32
21	10.28	13.24	16.34	20.34	24.93	29.62	32.67	35.48	38.93	46.80
22	10.98	14.04	17.24	21.34	26.04	30.81	33.92	36.78	40.29	48.27
23	11.69	14.85	18.14	22.34	27.14	32.01	35.17	38.08	41.64	49.73
24	12.40	15.66	19.04	23.34	28.24	33.20	36.42	39.36	42.98	51.18
25	13.12	16.47	19.94	24.34	29.34	34.38	37.65	40.65	44.31	32.62
26	13.84	17.29	20.84	25.34	30.43	35.56	38.89	41.92	45.64	54.05
27	14.57	18.11	21.75	26.34	31.53	36.74	40.11	43.19	46.96	55.48
28	15.31	18.94	22.66	27.34	32.62	37.92	41.34	44.46	48.28	56.89
29	16.05	19.77	23.57	28.34	33.71	39.09	42.56	45.72	49.59	58.30
30	16.79	20.60	24.48	29.34	34.80	40.26	43.77	46.98	50.89	59.70
40	24.43	29.05	33.66	39.34	45.62	51.80	55.76	59.34	63.69	73.40
50	32.36	37.69	42.94	49.33	56.33	63.17	67.50	71.42	76.15	86.66
60	40.48	46.46	52.29	59.33	66.98	74.40	79.08	83.30	88.38	99.61
70	48.76	55.33	61.70	69.33	77.58	85.53	90.53	95.02	100.42	112.32
80	57.15	64.28	71.14	79.33	88.13	96.58	101.88	106.63	112.33	124.84
90	65.65	73.29	80.62	89.33	98.64	107.56	113.14	118.14	124.12	137.21
100	74.22	82.36	90.13	99.33	109.14	118.50	124.34	129.56	135.81	149.45

Condensed from Table 8 of Pearson, E. S. and Hartley, H. O. (1966) *Biometrika Tables for Statisticians,* 3rd Edn. Cambridge: Cambridge University Press.

Table A3 Percentage points of the Student t-distribution

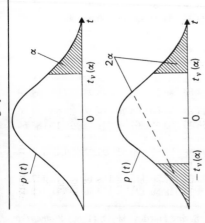

The percentage point, $t_\nu(\alpha)$, beyond which lies $100\alpha\%$ of the probability, is tabulated for various values of ν and α. The distribution is symmetric about $t_\nu(0.50) = 0$ so that $t_\nu(\alpha) = -t_\nu(1-\alpha)$.

The percentage point, $t_\nu(\alpha)$, is also tabulated for various values of ν and 2α. Consideration is given here to both tails of the distribution, $100\alpha\%$ of the total probability lying beyond $t_\nu(\alpha)$ and $100\alpha\%$ of the total probability lying below $-t_\nu(\alpha)$.

DF ν / α / 2α	0.45 / 0.90	0.40 / 0.80	0.35 / 0.70	0.30 / 0.60	0.25 / 0.50	0.20 / 0.40	0.15 / 0.30	0.10 / 0.20	0.05 / 0.10	0.025 / 0.050	0.010 / 0.020	0.005 / 0.010	0.0005 / 0.0010
1	0.158	0.325	0.510	0.727	1.000	1.376	1.963	3.078	6.314	12.706	31.821	63.657	636.619
2	0.142	0.289	0.445	0.617	0.816	1.061	1.386	1.886	2.920	4.303	6.965	9.925	31.598
3	0.137	0.277	0.424	0.584	0.765	0.978	1.250	1.638	2.353	3.182	4.541	5.841	12.924
4	0.134	0.271	0.414	0.569	0.741	0.941	1.190	1.533	2.132	2.776	3.747	4.604	8.610
5	0.132	0.267	0.408	0.559	0.727	0.920	1.156	1.476	2.015	2.571	3.365	4.032	6.869
6	0.131	0.265	0.404	0.553	0.718	0.906	1.134	1.440	1.943	2.447	3.143	3.707	5.959
7	0.130	0.263	0.402	0.549	0.711	0.896	1.119	1.415	1.895	2.365	2.998	3.499	5.408
8	0.130	0.262	0.399	0.546	0.706	0.889	1.108	1.397	1.860	2.306	2.896	3.355	5.041
9	0.129	0.261	0.398	0.543	0.703	0.883	1.100	1.383	1.833	2.262	2.821	3.250	4.781
10	0.129	0.260	0.397	0.542	0.700	0.879	1.093	1.372	1.812	2.228	2.764	3.169	4.587

11	0.129	0.260	0.396	0.540	0.697	0.876	1.088	1.363	1.796	2.201	2.718	3.106	4.437
12	0.128	0.259	0.395	0.539	0.695	0.873	1.083	1.356	1.782	2.179	2.681	3.055	4.318
13	0.128	0.259	0.394	0.538	0.694	0.870	1.079	1.350	1.771	2.160	2.650	3.012	4.221
14	0.128	0.258	0.393	0.537	0.692	0.868	1.076	1.345	1.761	2.145	2.624	2.977	4.140
15	0.128	0.258	0.393	0.536	0.691	0.866	1.074	1.341	1.753	2.131	2.602	2.947	4.073
16	0.128	0.258	0.392	0.535	0.690	0.865	1.071	1.337	1.746	2.120	2.583	2.921	4.015
17	0.128	0.257	0.392	0.534	0.689	0.863	1.069	1.333	1.740	2.110	2.567	2.898	3.965
18	0.127	0.257	0.392	0.534	0.688	0.862	1.067	1.330	1.734	2.101	2.552	2.878	3.922
19	0.127	0.257	0.391	0.533	0.688	0.861	1.066	1.328	1.729	2.093	2.539	2.861	3.883
20	0.127	0.257	0.391	0.533	0.687	0.860	1.064	1.325	1.725	2.086	2.528	2.845	3.850
21	0.127	0.257	0.391	0.532	0.686	0.859	1.063	1.323	1.721	2.080	2.518	2.831	3.819
22	0.127	0.256	0.390	0.532	0.686	0.858	1.061	1.321	1.717	2.074	2.508	2.819	3.792
23	0.127	0.256	0.390	0.532	0.685	0.858	1.060	1.319	1.714	2.069	2.500	2.807	3.767
24	0.127	0.256	0.390	0.531	0.685	0.857	1.059	1.318	1.711	2.064	2.492	2.797	3.745
25	0.127	0.256	0.390	0.531	0.684	0.856	1.058	1.316	1.708	2.060	2.485	2.787	3.725
26	0.127	0.256	0.390	0.531	0.684	0.856	1.058	1.315	1.706	2.056	2.479	2.779	3.707
27	0.127	0.256	0.389	0.531	0.684	0.855	1.057	1.314	1.703	2.052	2.473	2.771	3.690
28	0.127	0.256	0.389	0.530	0.683	0.855	1.056	1.313	1.701	2.048	2.467	2.763	3.674
29	0.127	0.256	0.389	0.530	0.683	0.854	1.055	1.311	1.699	2.045	2.462	2.756	3.659
30	0.127	0.256	0.389	0.530	0.683	0.854	1.055	1.310	1.697	2.042	2.457	2.750	3.646
40	0.126	0.255	0.388	0.529	0.681	0.851	1.050	1.303	1.684	2.021	2.423	2.704	3.551
50	0.126	0.255	0.388	0.528	0.679	0.849	1.047	1.299	1.676	2.009	2.403	2.678	3.497
100	0.126	0.254	0.386	0.526	0.677	0.845	1.042	1.290	1.660	1.984	2.364	2.626	3.391
200	0.126	0.254	0.386	0.525	0.676	0.843	1.039	1.286	1.653	1.972	2.345	2.601	3.340
∞	0.126	0.253	0.385	0.524	0.674	0.842	1.036	1.282	1.645	1.960	2.326	2.576	3.291

Extracted from *Documenta Geigy Scientific Tables*, 7th Edn., Basle, 1970. Courtesy CIBA GEIGY Limited, Basle, Switzerland.

Table A4 Percentage points of the F-distribution

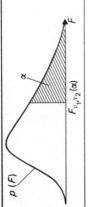

The percentage point $F_{v_1, v_2}(\alpha)$, beyond which lies $100\alpha\%$ of the total probability, is tabulated for various values of v_1 and v_2 and for $\alpha = 0.05, 0.01, 0.001$.

DF denominator, v_2	α	1	2	3	4	5	6	7	8	9	10	20	30	60	120	∞
								DF for numerator, v_1								
1	$\alpha = 0.05$	161.4	199.5	215.7	224.6	230.2	234.0	236.8	238.9	240.5	241.9	248.0	250.1	252.2	253.3	254.3
	$\alpha = 0.01$	4052	5000	5403	5625	5764	5859	5928	5981	6022	6056	6209	6261	6313	6339	6366
	$\alpha = 0.001$	4053*	5000*	5404*	5625*	5764*	5859*	5929*	5981*	6023*	6056*	6209*	6261*	6313*	6340*	6366*
2		18.51	19.00	19.16	19.25	19.30	19.33	19.35	19.37	19.38	19.40	19.45	19.46	19.48	19.49	19.50
		98.50	99.00	99.17	99.25	99.30	99.33	99.36	99.37	99.39	99.40	99.45	99.47	99.48	99.49	99.50
		998.5	999.0	999.2	999.2	999.3	999.3	999.4	999.4	999.4	999.4	999.4	999.5	999.5	999.5	999.5
3		10.13	9.55	9.28	9.12	9.01	8.94	8.89	8.85	8.81	8.79	8.66	8.62	8.57	8.55	8.53
		34.12	30.82	29.46	28.71	28.24	27.91	27.67	27.49	27.35	27.23	26.69	26.50	26.32	26.22	26.13
		167.0	148.5	141.1	137.1	134.6	132.8	131.6	130.6	129.9	129.2	126.4	125.4	124.5	124.0	123.5
4		7.71	6.94	6.59	6.39	6.26	6.16	6.09	6.04	6.00	5.96	5.80	5.75	5.69	5.66	5.63
		21.20	18.00	16.69	15.98	15.52	15.21	14.98	14.80	14.66	14.55	14.02	13.84	13.65	13.56	13.46
		74.14	61.25	56.18	53.44	51.71	50.53	49.66	49.00	48.47	48.05	46.10	45.43	44.75	44.40	44.05
5		6.61	5.79	5.41	5.19	5.05	4.95	4.88	4.82	4.77	4.74	4.56	4.50	4.43	4.40	4.36
		16.26	13.27	12.06	11.39	10.97	10.67	10.46	10.29	10.16	10.05	9.55	9.38	9.20	9.11	9.02
		47.18	37.12	33.20	31.09	29.75	28.84	28.16	27.64	27.24	26.92	25.39	24.87	24.33	24.06	23.79

6	5.99	5.14	4.76	4.53	4.39	4.28	4.21	4.15	4.10	4.06	3.87	3.81	3.74	3.70	3.67
	13.75	10.92	9.78	9.15	8.75	8.47	8.26	8.10	7.98	7.87	7.40	7.23	7.06	6.97	6.88
	35.51	27.00	23.70	21.92	20.81	20.03	19.46	19.03	18.69	18.41	17.12	16.67	16.21	15.99	15.75
7	5.59	4.74	4.35	4.12	3.97	3.87	3.79	3.73	3.68	3.64	3.44	3.38	3.30	3.27	3.23
	12.25	9.55	8.45	7.85	7.46	7.19	6.99	6.84	6.72	6.62	6.16	5.99	5.82	5.74	5.65
	29.25	21.69	18.77	17.19	16.21	15.52	15.02	14.63	14.33	14.08	12.93	12.53	12.12	11.91	11.70
8	5.32	4.46	4.07	3.84	3.69	3.58	3.50	3.44	3.39	3.35	3.15	3.08	3.01	2.97	2.93
	11.26	8.65	7.59	7.01	6.63	6.37	6.18	6.03	5.91	5.81	5.36	5.20	5.03	4.95	4.86
	25.42	18.49	15.83	14.39	13.49	12.86	12.40	12.04	11.77	11.54	10.48	10.11	9.73	9.53	9.33
9	5.12	4.26	3.86	3.63	3.48	3.37	3.29	3.23	3.18	3.14	2.94	2.86	2.79	2.75	2.71
	10.56	8.02	6.99	6.42	6.06	5.80	5.61	5.47	5.35	5.26	4.81	4.65	4.48	4.40	4.31
	22.86	16.39	13.90	12.56	11.71	11.13	10.70	10.37	10.11	9.89	8.90	8.55	8.19	8.00	7.81
10	4.96	4.10	3.71	3.48	3.33	3.22	3.14	3.07	3.02	2.98	2.77	2.70	2.62	2.58	2.54
	10.04	7.56	6.55	5.99	5.64	5.39	5.20	5.06	4.94	4.85	4.41	4.25	4.08	4.00	3.91
	21.04	14.91	12.55	11.28	10.48	9.92	9.52	9.20	8.96	8.75	7.80	7.47	7.12	6.94	6.76
11	4.84	3.98	3.59	3.36	3.20	3.09	3.01	2.95	2.90	2.85	2.65	2.57	2.49	2.45	2.40
	9.65	7.21	6.22	5.67	5.32	5.07	4.89	4.74	4.63	4.54	4.10	3.94	3.78	3.69	3.60
	19.69	13.81	11.56	10.35	9.58	9.05	8.66	8.35	8.12	7.92	7.01	6.68	6.35	6.17	6.00
12	4.75	3.89	3.49	3.26	3.11	3.00	2.91	2.85	2.80	2.75	2.54	2.47	2.38	2.34	2.30
	9.33	6.93	5.95	5.41	5.06	4.82	4.64	4.50	4.39	4.30	3.86	3.70	3.54	3.45	3.36
	18.64	12.97	10.80	9.63	8.89	8.38	8.00	7.71	7.48	7.29	6.40	6.09	5.76	5.59	5.42
13	4.67	3.81	3.41	3.18	3.03	2.92	2.83	2.77	2.71	2.67	2.46	2.38	2.30	2.25	2.21
	9.07	6.70	5.74	5.21	4.86	4.62	4.44	4.30	4.19	4.10	3.66	3.51	3.34	3.25	3.17
	17.81	12.31	10.21	9.07	8.35	7.86	7.49	7.21	6.98	6.80	5.93	5.63	5.30	5.14	4.97
14	4.60	3.74	3.34	3.11	2.96	2.85	2.76	2.70	2.65	2.60	2.39	2.31	2.22	2.18	2.13
	8.86	6.51	5.56	5.04	4.69	4.46	4.28	4.14	4.03	3.94	3.51	3.35	3.18	3.09	3.00
	17.14	11.78	9.73	8.62	7.92	7.43	7.08	6.80	6.58	6.40	5.56	5.25	4.94	4.77	4.60

Table A4 *continued*

DF denominator, v_2	α	1	2	3	4	5	6	7	8	9	10	20	30	60	120	∞
							DF for numerator, v_1									
15	$\alpha = 0.05$	4.54	3.68	3.29	3.06	2.90	2.79	2.71	2.64	2.59	2.54	2.33	2.25	2.16	2.11	2.07
	$\alpha = 0.01$	8.68	6.36	5.42	4.89	4.56	4.32	4.14	4.00	3.89	3.80	3.37	3.21	3.05	2.96	2.87
	$\alpha = 0.001$	16.59	11.34	9.34	8.25	7.57	7.09	6.74	6.47	6.26	6.08	5.25	4.95	4.64	4.47	4.31
16		4.49	3.63	3.24	3.01	2.85	2.74	2.66	2.59	2.54	2.49	2.28	2.19	2.11	2.06	2.01
		8.53	6.23	5.29	4.77	4.44	4.20	4.03	3.89	3.78	3.69	3.26	3.10	2.93	2.84	2.75
		16.12	10.97	9.00	7.94	7.27	6.81	6.46	6.19	5.98	5.81	4.99	4.70	4.39	4.23	4.06
17		4.45	3.59	3.20	2.96	2.81	2.70	2.61	2.55	2.49	2.45	2.23	2.15	2.06	2.01	1.96
		8.40	6.11	5.18	4.67	4.34	4.10	3.93	3.79	3.68	3.59	3.16	3.00	2.83	2.75	2.65
		15.72	10.66	8.73	7.68	7.02	6.56	6.22	5.96	5.75	5.58	4.78	4.48	4.18	4.02	3.85
18		4.41	3.55	3.16	2.93	2.77	2.66	2.58	2.51	2.46	2.41	2.19	2.11	2.02	1.97	1.92
		8.29	6.01	5.09	4.58	4.25	4.01	3.84	3.71	3.60	3.51	3.08	2.92	2.75	2.66	2.57
		15.38	10.39	8.49	7.46	6.81	6.35	6.02	5.76	5.56	5.39	4.59	4.30	4.00	3.84	3.67
19		4.38	3.52	3.13	2.90	2.74	2.63	2.54	2.48	2.42	2.38	2.16	2.07	1.98	1.93	1.88
		8.18	5.93	5.01	4.50	4.17	3.94	3.77	3.63	3.52	3.43	3.00	2.84	2.67	2.58	2.49
		15.08	10.16	8.28	7.26	6.62	6.18	5.85	5.59	5.39	5.22	4.43	4.14	3.84	3.68	3.51
20		4.35	3.49	3.10	2.87	2.71	2.60	2.51	2.45	2.39	2.35	2.12	2.04	1.95	1.90	1.84
		8.10	5.85	4.94	4.43	4.10	3.87	3.70	3.56	3.46	3.37	2.94	2.78	2.61	2.52	2.42
		14.82	9.95	8.10	7.10	6.46	6.02	5.69	5.44	5.24	5.08	4.29	4.00	3.70	3.54	3.38
25		4.24	3.39	2.99	2.76	2.60	2.49	2.40	2.34	2.28	2.24	2.01	1.92	1.82	1.77	1.71
		7.77	5.57	4.68	4.18	3.85	3.63	3.46	3.32	3.22	3.13	2.70	2.54	2.36	2.27	2.17
		13.88	9.22	7.45	6.49	5.88	5.46	5.15	4.91	4.71	4.56	3.79	3.52	3.22	3.06	2.89

30	4.17	3.32	2.92	2.69	2.53	2.42	2.33	2.27	2.21	2.16	1.93	1.84	1.74	1.68	1.62
	7.56	5.39	4.51	4.02	3.70	3.47	3.30	3.17	3.07	2.98	2.55	2.39	2.21	2.11	2.01
	13.29	8.77	7.05	6.12	5.53	5.12	4.82	4.58	4.39	4.24	3.49	3.22	2.92	2.76	2.59
40	4.08	3.23	2.84	2.61	2.45	2.34	2.25	2.18	2.12	2.08	1.84	1.74	1.64	1.58	1.51
	7.31	5.18	4.31	3.83	3.51	3.29	3.12	2.99	2.89	2.80	2.37	2.20	2.02	1.92	1.80
	12.61	8.25	6.60	5.70	5.13	4.73	4.44	4.21	4.02	3.87	3.15	2.87	2.57	2.41	2.23
60	4.00	3.15	2.76	2.53	2.37	2.25	2.17	2.10	2.04	1.99	1.75	1.65	1.53	1.47	1.39
	7.08	4.98	4.13	3.65	3.34	3.12	2.95	2.82	2.72	2.63	2.20	2.03	1.84	1.73	1.60
	11.97	7.76	6.17	5.31	4.76	4.37	4.09	3.87	3.69	3.54	2.83	2.55	2.25	2.08	1.89
120	3.92	3.07	2.68	2.45	2.29	2.17	2.09	2.02	1.96	1.91	1.66	1.55	1.43	1.35	1.25
	6.85	4.79	3.95	3.48	3.17	2.96	2.79	2.66	2.56	2.47	2.03	1.86	1.66	1.53	1.38
	11.38	7.32	5.79	4.95	4.42	4.04	3.77	3.55	3.38	3.24	2.53	2.26	1.95	1.76	1.54
∞	3.88	3.00	2.60	2.37	2.21	2.10	2.01	1.94	1.88	1.83	1.57	1.46	1.32	1.22	1.00
	6.63	4.61	3.78	3.32	3.02	2.80	2.64	2.51	2.41	2.32	1.88	1.70	1.47	1.32	1.00
	10.83	6.91	5.42	4.62	4.10	3.74	3.47	3.27	3.10	2.96	2.27	1.99	1.66	1.45	1.00

*Multiply these entries by 100.

Condensed from Table 18 of Pearson, E. S. and Hartley, H. O. (1966) *Biometrika Tables for Statisticians*. 3rd Edn. Cambridge: Cambridge University Press.

Appendix

Table A5 Values of the correlation coefficient, r, at different levels of significance when testing H_0: $\rho = 0$. For a *two-tailed* test, significance is achieved at the specified level if the absolute value of the sample correlation coefficient based on n pairs of observations exceeds the tabulated value ($\nu = n-2$). For a one-tailed test, the significance level is halved

DF, ν	2α 0.05	0.01	0.001	DF, ν	2α 0.05	0.01	0.001
1	0.9969	0.9999	1.0000	21	0.4132	0.5256	0.6402
2	0.9500	0.9900	0.9990	22	0.4044	0.5151	0.6287
3	0.8783	0.9587	0.9911	23	0.3961	0.5052	0.6177
4	0.8114	0.9172	0.9741	24	0.3882	0.4958	0.6073
5	0.7545	0.8745	0.9509	25	0.3809	0.4869	0.5974
6	0.7067	0.8343	0.9249	26	0.3739	0.4785	0.5880
7	0.6664	0.7977	0.8983	27	0.3673	0.4705	0.5790
8	0.6319	0.7646	0.8721	28	0.3610	0.4629	0.5703
9	0.6021	0.7348	0.8471	29	0.3550	0.4556	0.5620
10	0.5760	0.7079	0.8233	30	0.3494	0.4487	0.5541
11	0.5529	0.6835	0.8010	35	0.3246	0.4182	0.5189
12	0.5324	0.6614	0.7800	40	0.3044	0.3932	0.4896
13	0.5139	0.6411	0.7604	45	0.2875	0.3721	0.4647
14	0.4973	0.6226	0.7419	50	0.2732	0.3541	0.4433
15	0.4821	0.6055	0.7247	60	0.2500	0.3248	0.4079
16	0.4683	0.5897	0.7084	70	0.2319	0.3017	0.3798
17	0.4555	0.5751	0.6932	80	0.2172	0.2830	0.3569
18	0.4438	0.5614	0.6788	90	0.2050	0.2673	0.3376
19	0.4329	0.5487	0.6652	100	0.1946	0.2540	0.3211
20	0.4227	0.5368	0.6524	200	0.1381	0.1809	0.2299

H_0: $\rho = 0 \equiv H_0$: $\beta = 0$ from which $r\sqrt{n-2}/\sqrt{1-r^2}$ is distributed as t_ν.
Table A5 is constructed from this quotient.
Extracted from *Documenta Geigy Scientific Tables*, 7th Edn., Basle, 1970. Courtesy CIBA-GEIGY Limited. Basle: Switzerland.

Table A6 Wilcoxon rank sum test. Critical values of T_{17} at different levels of significance ($2\alpha = 0.05, 0.01, 0.001$) when $n_1 + n_2 \leq 30$. n_1 and n_2 are the numbers of observations in the two samples. If the samples are unequal in size, n_1 refers to the smaller. For a *two-tailed* test, significance is achieved at the specified level if T_{17C} is less than or equal to the tabulated critical value

n_2	2α	n_1 2	3	4	5	6	7	8	9	10	11	12	13	14	15
4	0.05			10											
5	0.05		6	11	17										
	0.01				15										
6	0.05		7	12	18	26									
	0.01			10	16	23									
7	0.05		7	13	20	27	36								
	0.01			10	17	24	32								
	0.001						28								
8	0.05	3	8	14	21	29	38	49							
	0.01			11	17	25	34	43							
	0.001				21	29	38								
9	0.05	3	8	15	22	31	40	51	63						
	0.01		6	11	18	26	35	45	56						
	0.001			15	22	30	40	50							
10	0.05	3	9	15	23	32	42	53	65	78					
	0.01		6	12	19	27	37	47	58	71					
	0.001			15	23	31	41	52	63						
11	0.05	4	9	16	24	34	44	55	68	81	96				
	0.01		6	12	20	28	38	48	61	74	87				
	0.001				16	23	32	42	53	65	78				
12	0.05	4	10	17	26	35	46	58	71	85	99	115			
	0.01		7	13	21	30	40	51	63	76	90	106			
	0.001				16	24	33	43	55	67	81	95			
13	0.05	4	10	18	27	37	48	60	73	88	103	119	137		
	0.01		7	14	22	31	41	53	65	79	93	109	125		
	0.001			10	17	25	34	45	56	69	83	98	114		
14	0.05	4	11	19	28	38	50	63	76	91	106	123	141	160	
	0.01		7	14	22	32	43	54	67	81	96	112	129	147	
	0.001			10	17	26	35	46	58	71	85	100	116	134	
15	0.05	4	11	20	29	40	52	65	79	94	110	127	145	164	185
	0.01		8	15	23	33	44	56	70	84	99	115	133	151	171
	0.001			10	18	26	36	47	60	73	87	103	119	137	156
16	0.05	4	12	21	31	42	54	67	82	97	114	131	150	169	
	0.01		8	15	24	34	46	58	72	86	102	119	137	155	
	0.001		11	18	27	37	49	61	75	90	105	122	140		

Table A6 *continued*

n_2	2α	n_1													
		2	3	4	5	6	7	8	9	10	11	12	13	14	15
17	0.05	5	12	21	32	43	56	70	84	100	117	135	154		
	0.01		8	16	25	36	47	60	74	89	105	122	140		
	0.001			11	19	28	38	50	63	77	92	108	125		
18	0.05	5	13	22	33	45	58	72	87	103	121	139			
	0.01		8	16	26	37	49	62	76	92	108	125			
	0.001			11	19	29	39	51	65	79	94	111			
19	0.05	5	13	23	34	46	60	74	90	107	124				
	0.01	3	9	17	27	38	50	64	78	94	111				
	0.001			12	20	29	41	53	66	81	97				
20	0.05	5	14	24	35	48	62	77	93	110					
	0.01	3	9	18	28	39	52	66	81	97					
	0.001			12	20	30	42	54	68	83					
21	0.05	6	14	25	37	50	64	79	95						
	0.01	3	9	18	29	40	53	68	83						
	0.001		6	12	21	31	43	56	70						
22	0.05	6	15	26	38	51	66	82							
	0.01	3	10	19	29	42	55	70							
	0.001		6	13	21	32	44	57							
23	0.05	6	15	27	39	53	68								
	0.01	3	10	19	30	43	57								
	0.001		6	13	22	33	45								
24	0.05	6	16	28	40	55									
	0.01	3	10	20	31	44									
	0.001		6	13	23	34									
25	0.05	6	16	28	42										
	0.01	3	11	20	32										
	0.001		6	14	23										
26	0.05	6	17	29											
	0.01	3	11	21											
	0.001		6	14											
27	0.05	7	17												
	0.01	4	11												
	0.001		7												
28	0.05	7													
	0.01	4													

Reproduced from White, C. (1952) The use of ranks in a test of significance for comparing two treatments. *Biometrics*, **8,** 33–41. With permission of the Biometric Society.

Table A7 Wilcoxon signed rank test. Critical values of T_{19} at different levels of significance ($2\alpha = 0.05$, 0.01); n is the number of non-zero differences. For a *two-tailed* test, significance is achieved at the specified level if T_{19C} is less than or equal to the tabulated critical value.

	2α				2α	
n	0.05	0.01		n	0.05	0.01
6	0	—		16	30	20
7	2	—		17	35	23
8	4	0		18	40	28
9	6	2		19	46	32
10	8	3		20	52	38
11	11	5		21	59	43
12	14	7		22	66	49
13	17	10		23	73	55
14	21	13		24	81	61
15	25	16		25	89	68

Adapted from Table I of Wilcoxon, F. (1949) *Some Rapid Approximate Statistical Procedures*. New York: American Cyanamid Company.

Table A8 Random numbers

---

02 34 64 55 31	40 75 30 74 05	93 16 38 20 19	18 13 50 71 57	23 46 29 66 39
30 01 08 22 67	48 62 15 59 28	57 98 65 05 39	24 06 47 20 70	00 43 17 47 14
28 64 43 25 78	88 72 81 32 92	73 09 73 72 17	83 60 65 09 76	93 55 82 04 93
66 64 84 88 87	28 85 18 36 89	06 79 83 16 27	64 50 82 70 23	74 20 89 62 74
10 05 22 16 92	39 82 97 42 10	35 00 85 22 45	11 42 81 84 19	67 45 51 41 73
27 16 61 45 62	72 32 19 95 37	44 24 74 92 82	13 92 55 05 62	91 36 80 87 99
70 36 69 03 79	02 72 63 12 50	25 78 36 90 50	76 71 09 47 40	26 09 80 81 72
50 64 26 76 11	77 27 73 92 45	60 58 93 60 62	76 33 77 65 35	22 60 74 14 12
27 76 91 93 45	10 19 83 99 45	09 43 76 92 79	71 49 96 71 49	63 23 87 66 03
76 84 07 94 27	66 11 88 78 46	10 74 01 26 40	00 28 52 67 66	07 78 48 74 79
03 57 30 84 94	80 21 66 04 15	14 94 04 41 98	87 27 41 58 12	01 30 87 67 72
19 50 86 95 50	64 75 71 30 87	05 62 78 64 78	29 78 72 33 45	37 31 28 75 75
68 42 14 84 70	34 61 25 05 16	11 66 32 93 01	74 19 14 31 56	92 62 26 06 69
76 01 53 35 62	02 14 55 05 94	36 80 53 67 95	09 29 64 74 36	74 49 84 66 16
56 02 13 93 21	84 52 14 96 06	34 35 09 46 77	21 77 64 97 62	97 74 58 93 15
71 94 78 09 08	32 30 28 22 53	90 94 03 65 64	42 85 95 60 00	16 32 99 35 14
00 90 36 87 69	89 17 23 30 00	94 86 83 89 60	22 35 14 05 57	09 26 73 30 34
65 84 40 62 81	16 01 37 11 31	71 68 44 96 29	05 10 12 45 72	92 05 14 30 82
71 05 60 48 65	24 45 23 37 54	06 90 87 84 44	36 22 56 20 97	60 92 47 83 11
22 24 63 02 76	41 18 55 83 44	13 33 23 34 24	04 33 27 82 66	86 36 50 45 77
04 22 76 32 80	88 74 19 56 17	07 36 17 23 29	04 48 96 60 01	66 12 41 35 83
86 72 93 83 63	34 75 50 54 02	26 49 92 91 86	51 21 84 81 49	10 35 09 87 75
96 50 84 02 77	10 25 06 63 22	10 45 44 69 88	87 57 98 33 09	48 16 44 72 22
35 63 40 69 52	74 30 43 82 39	86 09 74 30 59	60 47 08 47 41	62 65 44 79 77
77 34 40 77 65	83 23 41 44 28	93 16 21 40 76	43 07 44 74 91	96 09 02 52 03
23 01 71 61 37	30 99 22 70 87	30 99 22 70 87	90 76 31 69 17	66 50 09 39 49
31 96 19 68 07	01 08 54 20 73	01 08 54 20 73	70 16 32 99 69	60 26 04 43 61
11 13 63 24 47	09 74 65 74 23	09 74 65 74 23	67 62 23 74 57	88 45 75 23 37
01 04 41 35 27	64 93 32 15 29	64 93 32 15 29	44 48 76 58 68	42 03 95 62 67
81 97 31 17 89	79 01 62 98 46	79 01 62 98 46	95 31 96 60 18	04 23 06 30 27
50 73 06 39 73	31 17 08 73 17	82 25 28 53 13	13 89 23 88 30	63 58 27 96 73
45 80 89 69 92	55 94 22 18 82	40 01 78 50 05	99 69 41 08 09	37 55 01 61 59
71 82 70 81 33	98 20 37 98 58	82 32 45 29 17	34 69 12 10 65	48 98 02 70 73
22 02 66 22 47	74 13 55 59 05	59 17 16 04 51	51 39 51 55 05	68 88 09 80 01
68 45 81 50 20	76 25 27 76 48	69 12 97 38 36	05 07 18 99 83	57 03 21 00 04
03 03 51 04 64	13 96 43 74 57	46 78 08 83 74	01 69 74 69 21	80 15 88 25 76
50 70 60 26 87	81 22 51 33 44	91 84 81 45 03	26 87 94 08 38	21 32 43 02 37
57 00 77 75 33	99 53 56 05 34	51 67 04 69 88	28 42 29 46 50	69 41 29 86 14
90 51 71 24 69	45 32 39 84 51	65 12 14 15 85	34 52 03 81 54	30 33 02 87 68
75 75 65 95 33	23 72 86 82 80	32 86 45 62 13	19 39 82 43 20	14 06 77 39 33
75 98 56 87 90	71 01 76 65 72	95 50 69 19 43	31 97 79 48 40	04 29 97 46 03
19 43 10 64 11	67 75 19 59 29	46 46 26 90 30	13 24 91 13 98	50 02 32 24 48
86 33 76 92 25	44 37 06 75 56	48 74 43 37 80	32 92 85 43 29	19 33 57 28 58
12 74 95 04 75	60 11 36 64 61	36 33 29 39 22	43 21 04 30 14	23 52 06 74 24
75 06 09 85 74	57 96 27 48 51	63 43 33 83 04	10 53 89 14 98	62 91 46 48 76

References

Anderson, J. A. (1972) Separate sample logistic discrimination. *Biometrika*, **59**, 19–34.

Anderson, S., Auquier, A., Hauck, W. W., Oakes, D., Vandaele, W. and Weisberg, H. I. (1980) *Statistical Methods for Comparative Studies*. Chichester: Wiley.

Armitage, P. (1987) *Statistical Methods in Medical Research*, 2nd Edn. Oxford: Blackwell Scientific Publications.

Armitage, P. (1975) *Sequential Medical Trials*, 2nd Edn. Oxford: Blackwell Scientific Publications.

Breslow, N. E. and Day, N. E. (1980) *Statistical Methods in Cancer Research. Volume I—The Analysis of Case-control Studies*. Lyon: IARC.

British Medical Association (1980) *The Handbook of Medical Ethics*. London: British Medical Association.

Cockburn, F., Belton, N. R., Purvis, R. J. *et al.* (1980) Maternal vitamin D intake and mineral metabolism in mothers and their newborn infants. *Br. Med. J.*, **281**, 11–14.

Colditz, G. A., Stampfer, M. J., Willett, W. C. *et al.* (1986) A prospective study of parental history of myocardial infarction and coronary heart disease in women. *Am. J. Epidemiol.*, **123**, 48–58.

Coloquhoun, D. (1971) *Lectures on Biostatistics*. Oxford: Oxford University Press.

Corridan, J., O'Regan, J. P. and O'Sullivan, D. J. (1977) Diabetes and appendicectomy: testing a hypothesis. *Brit. Med. J.*, **i**, 1135.

Colton, T. (1974) *Statistics in Medicine*. New York: Little, Brown and Co.

Cox, D. R. (1958) *Planning of Experiments*. New York: Wiley.

Dawber, T. R., Meadors, G. F. and Moore, F. E. Jr. (1951) Epidemiological approaches to heart disease: the Framingham Study. *Am. J. Public Health*, **41**, 279–286.

Documenta Geigy (1970) *Scientific Tables*, 7th Edn. Basle.

Draper, N. R. and Smith, H. (1981) *Applied Regression Analysis*, 2nd Edn. Chichester: Wiley.

Fisher, R. A. and Yates, F. (1963) *Statistical Tables for Biological, Agricultural and Medical Research*, 6th Edn. Edinburgh: Oliver and Boyd.

Fleiss, J. (1981) *Statistical Methods for Rates and Proportions*, 2nd Edn. New York: Wiley.

Healy, M. J. R. and Osborn, J. (1986) *Manual of Medical Statistics. Volume II*. London: London School of Hygiene and Tropical Medicine.

Hill, A. B. (1971) *Principles of Medical Statistics*, 9th Edn. London: Lancet.

Hills, M. and Armitage, P. (1979) The two-period cross-over clinical trial. *Br. J. Clin. Pharmacol.*, **8**, 7–20.

Johansson, E., Pyrhönen, S. and Rostila, T. (1977) Warts and wart virus antibodies in patients with systemic lupus erythematosus. *Br. Med. J.*, **i**, 74–76.

Karlbfleish, J. D. and Prentice, R. L. (1980) *The Statistical Analysis of Failure Time Data*. Chichester: Wiley.

Kempthorne, O. (1952) *Design and Analysis of Experiments*. Chichester: Wiley.

Kendall, M. G. (1955) *Rank Correlation Methods*, 2nd Edn. London: Griffin.

Longley, D. and Shain, M. (1985) *Understanding Microcomputers*. London: Macmillan Press.

Macfarlane, P. W. (ed.) (1985) *Computer Techniques in Clinical Medicine*. London: Butterworths.

MacMahon, B. and Pugh, T. F. (1970) *Epidemiology: Principles and Methods*. New York: Little, Brown and Co.

Mantel, N. and Haenszel, W. (1959) Statistical analysis of data from retrospective studies of disease. *J. Nat. Cancer Inst.*, **22**, 719–748.

Markowe, H. L. J., Marmot, M. G., Shipley, M. J. *et al.* (1985) Fibrinogen: a possible link between social class and coronary heart disease. *Br. Med. J.*, **291**, 1312–1314.

Matthews, D. E. and Farewell, V. (1985) *Using and Understanding Medical Statistics*. Basel: Karger.

Medical Research Council (1963) Responsibility in investigations on human subjects. Annual Report, 1962–3, Cmnd 2382, HMSO, reprinted in *Br. Med. J.* (1964), **ii**, 178–180.

Miettinen, O. S. (1970) Estimation of relative risk from individually matched series. *Biometrics*, **26**, 75–86.

Oakes, D. (1983) Comparison of models for survival data. *Stat. Med.*, **2**, 305–311.

Osborn, J. F. (1975) A multiplicative model for the analysis of vital statistics rates. *J. R. Statist. Soc.* (C), **24**, 75–84.

Osborn, J. F. (1986) *Basic Statistical Methods for Epidemiological Studies*. London: London School of Hygiene and Tropical Medicine.

Pearson, E. S. and Hartley, H. O. (1966) *Biometrika Tables for Statisticians*, 3rd Edn. Cambridge: Cambridge University Press.

Peto, R., Pike, M. C., Armitage, P. *et al.* (1977) Design and analysis of randomised clinical trials requiring prolonged observation of each patient: II analysis and examples. *Br. J. Cancer*, **35**, 1–39.

Pocock, S. J. (1976) The combination of randomised and historical controls in clinical trials. *J. Chronic. Dis.*, **29**, 175–188.

Pocock, S. J. (1977) Group sequential methods in the design and analysis of clinical trials. *Biometrika*, **64**, 191–199.

Pocock, S. J. (1982) Interim analyses for randomised clinical trials: the group sequential approach. *Biometrics*, **38**, 153–162.

Pocock, S. J. (1983) *Clinical Trials. A Practical Approach*. Chichester: Wiley.

Report of the Sixty Plus Reinfarction Study Research Group (1980) A double-blind trial to assess long-term oral anticoagulant therapy in elderly patients after myocardial infarction. *Lancet*, **ii**, 989–994.

Royal College of Physicians (1967) Supervision of the ethics of clinical investigations in institutions. *Br. Med. J.*, **iii**, 429–430.

Schwartz, D., Flamart, R. and Lellouch, J. (1980) *Clinical Trials*. London: Academic Press.

Siegel, R. J. and Criley, J. M. (1985) Comparison of ventricular emptying with and without a pressure gradient in patients with hypertrophic cardiomyopathy. *Br. Heart J.*, **53**, 283–291.

Seigel, S. (1956) *Non-Parametric Statistics: for the Behavioural Sciences*. Tokyo: McGraw-Hill.

Shasby, D. M., Shope, T. C., Downs, H., Herrmann, K. L. and Polkowski, J. (1977) Epidemic measles in a highly vaccinated population. *N. Engl. J. Med.* **296**, 585–589.

Tuyns, A. J., Pequignot, G. and Jensen, O. M. (1977) Le cancer de l'oesophage en Ille-et-Vilaine en fonction des niveaux de consommation d'alcool et de tabac. *Bull. Cancer (Paris)*, **64**, 45–60.

Walker, S. H. and Duncan, D. B. (1967) Estimation of the probability of an event as a function of several independent variables. *Biometrika*, **54**, 167–179.

White, C. (1952) The use of ranks in a test of significance for comparing two treatments. *Biometrics*, **8**, 33–41.

Wilcoxon, F. (1949) *Some Rapid Approximate Statistical Procedures*. New York: Cyanamid Company.

Wildsmith, J. A. W. and Masson, A. H. B. (1974) Some effects of maintaining nitrogenation during anaesthesia. *Br. J. Anaesth.*, **46**, 680–684.

World Health Organization (1968) Principles for the clinical evaluation of drugs. *Tech. Rep. Ser. Wld. Hlth. Org.*, No. **403**.

World Medical Association (1964) Declaration of Helsinki. *Br. Med. J.*, **ii**, 177.

Index